# TRIAGE

## problem-oriented sorting of patients

Donald M. Vickery, M.D.

Health Services Director
Reston-Georgetown Medical Center
Reston, Virginia

Robert J. Brady Company
*A Prentice-Hall Company*
Bowie, Maryland 20715

# CONTENTS

# PREFACE

A basic problem in treating patients is assigning priorities to patients seeking medical care. Clearly it is impossible to provide immediate access to a physician for every patient. It is equally clear that, while every patient's problem does not require immediate attention, delay in the treatment of a patient who does have an emergent condition is undesirable and may result in tragedy. Perhaps the most vivid example of the need to decide who should be seen first is the military field hospital faced with mass battle casualties. It was in this setting that the term *triage* was first used to describe the life and death decisions that had to be made about the order in which soldiers would be treated.

Today *triage* is used to indicate the process by which patients requesting medical care are directed to medical providers in a medical center, outpatient department, or emergency room. While not as dramatic as in the setting of the battlefield, triage is just as necessary and may be a good deal more complicated. These triage decisions involve not only the question of when a patient will be seen but also where he will be seen and by whom. The range of possible answers to these questions has increased as the health care delivery has become more sophisticated. For example, does the patient's problem require immediate attention or can it wait an hour, a day, a week, or a month? Should he see a generalist, surgeon, pediatrician, nurse practitioner, physician's assistant, or other health-care provider? Should the encounter take place in an emergency treatment room, an isolation room, or an examining room? These questions must be answered for patients having numerous medical problems. Emergency facilities are confronted with an especially wide range of problems and possible treatments, a situation which makes a reliable triage mechanism mandatory.

The burden of triage falls on nurses, receptionists, and other allied health personnel. Most often it is the nurse who must assume the responsibility of triage, a responsibility which sometimes is underestimated by other members of the health-care team. Effective triage is necessary if patients are to be cared for by the right provider, at the right time, and in the right place. The lack of effective triage results in confusion and extra effort. This, in turn, inevitably leads to dissatisfied patients and frustrated providers, as well as morbidity and mortality which could have been prevented by the timely intervention of an appropriate provider.

This manual describes a system based on a problem-oriented approach to the making of triage decisions. Since this system of efficient and effective triage can be easily learned and implemented, any medical center, outpatient department, or emergency room can benefit from its use, saving patient and provider time, appropriately using personnel and equipment, and, most important, preventing unnecessary morbidity and mortality.

I am deeply indebted to Drs. Kenneth Larsen, Michael Soper, and Peter Collis for their assistance in the preparation of this manual.

As is true in any area of medicine, the guidelines in this manual must be interpreted in the light of the circumstances surrounding each patient encounter; their use must have the approval of those ultimately responsible for the care of the patient. The author and publisher can take no responsibility for acts arising out of their use.

I would like to thank Kenneth T. Larsen, M.D., Michael R. Soper, M.D., Peter B. Collis, M.D., and Richard F. Staley, M.D. for their medical assistance and Jacqueline V. Mummert for her clerical assistance in preparing this manuscript for publication.

Donald M. Vickery, M.D.

The purpose of this triage system is to direct patients without appointments to the appropriate provider of medical services at an appropriate time. Its central element is a set of clinical algorithms that is used to train and guide the triage workers. Clinical algorithms are simply rules for solving clinical problems. Unfortunate and unnecessary confusion has arisen with respect to the nature and use of clinical algorithms. For this reason the term *algorithm* is avoided altogether in the body of the manual. However, *algorithm* may be substituted for *rule* throughout the text without changing its meaning, if so desired.

The above comments notwithstanding, it may be useful to mention briefly the algorithmic approach to the training of allied health personnel. This approach involves two techniques: algorithmic task analysis, a process of defining the rules (algorithms) by which a clinical task is performed, and algorithmic task-specific training, training primarily based on these algorithms. The primary advantage of these techniques is the creation of exceedingly efficient training programs. For example, Red Cross volunteers require only about six hours of classroom training prior to beginning work in triage. A secondary advantage is the possibility of producing an exceedingly detailed job description for these workers.

The triage system described in this manual is based upon a system developed by the Automated Military Outpatient System (AMOS) Project at Fort Belvoir, Virginia. Modifications of the Fort Belvoir system are currently used in several Army hospitals and in the Medical Centers of the Georgetown University Community Health Plan. Well over 300,000 patients have been triaged in the last four years using modifications of the AMOS system. In all cases triage has been performed by personnel who have not received extensive medical training. In the Army hospitals the triage workers are, for the most part, Red Cross volunteers; in the Georgetown plan the receptionists are utilized for the purpose of triage. The error rate in dispositions, as determined by chart audit at Fort Belvoir, is less than three percent.

## Philosophy of Triage

There are a number of principles in the design of the system that should be made clear. First, the triage manual is primarily a training and reference manual. It is not expected that this manual will be used during each and every patient encounter after the completion of the training phase. It is expected that, due to their frequent use, many of the rules in the manual will be memorized. The manual need be consulted only when there is some doubt concerning the rules. Second, the triage system makes dispositions, not diagnoses. A disposition includes the name of the medical provider the patient is to see, the time of the visit, and any patient instructions, laboratory studies, or vital signs. Thirdly, the system is quite conservative in its dispositions. That is, a reasonable possibility of a serious disease always takes precedence over a reasonable probability of a minor disease. This system is far more concerned with quickly identifying a possibly emergent condition than directing a patient with a stable condition to a specialist.

## Organization of this Triage Manual

The next section, "The Triage Encounter," contains the rules which govern the triage encounter and the use of the flowsheets. A clear understanding of these rules by both the triage worker and supervisor is absolutely necessary if correct and efficient triage decisions are to be made. The most serious errors in triage almost inevitably result from neglect or misunderstanding of this section. The section also contains a sample triage encounter to illustrate the rules of the encounter and the use of the flowsheets.

The rules that deal with individual complaints then follow. These rules are displayed as flowsheets. The flowsheet questions use concise language in order to make them suitable for use as a reference. Accompanying each flowsheet is documentation to help explain questions and their purpose. This documentation will be most helpful during the training phase. At the end of each group of flowsheets are Criteria for Disposition. These criteria characterize the patient population being directed to each disposition.

## Triage Dispositions and the Health-Care Setting

The triage dispositions given in the manual make certain assumptions concerning personnel and facilities. The patient and triage worker are assumed to be in face-to-face contact in a reception area, although the system may be adapted for use by telephone (see the following discussion of system adaptation). The triage worker is called upon to. make certain observations but is not required to perform a physical examination or have the patient remove clothing.

The triage worker may direct patients to one of three types of rooms: an emergency treatment room, an isolation room, or an ordinary examining room. The emergency treatment room (ETR) is designated when there is the possibility of an emergency or when the special features of this room are required, as they are during the suturing of lacerations. The isolation room is used when certain infectious diseases are suspected; it has no special equipment. All other cases are seen in ordinary examining rooms. If the type of room is not given in the disposition, then the patient is to be seen in an ordinary examining room.

Available at all times to the triage worker are a physician and a physician's assistant. The physician is assumed to be a generalist competent to handle at least initial visits in virtually all areas of medicine. The vast majority of referrals to specialists will be made by the physician after the initial visit. Relatively few patients may be given a specialty appointment by the triage worker without consulting the physician.

The term *physician's assistant* is used generally and is meant to be interpreted in the broadest possible manner. The person assisting the physician may be a nurse practitioner, a Duke-type physician's assistant, a Medex, or some other type of a physician's assistant. The specific model of the physician's assistant (P.A.) used in development of the triage system is the AMOSIST developed by Project AMOS at Fort Belvoir. Disposi-tions are made to the P.A. in the expectation that the patient has an acute minor illness or that the P.A. may usefully gather clinical data for review by the physician.

There are four basic time periods for referral: STAT, Today, Appointment ASAP, and Routine Appointment. A disposition is made STAT if there is a possibility of an emergency. All STAT dispositions are made to the physician. Today disposi-tions form the vast majority; these patients are judged not to be emergencies but to need more detailed evaluation within twelve hours. When no time period is indicated for a disposition, the time period is Today; all dispositions to the P.A. are on this basis. If a patient is given an Appointment ASAP (as soon as possible) it is assumed that he or she will be seen within seven days of making that appointment. Routine Appointments are essentially at the convenience of patient and physician, al-though this is expected to be within a reasonable time, i.e., not more than two months.

By using the rules set forth in this manual, approximately fifty percent of patients will be directed to the physician's assistant. Less than five percent should receive appointments to specialists directly from the triage worker. The remainder will be referred to the physician, the majority to be seen on a Today basis. No more than five percent of the patients should be referred to the physician on a STAT basis.

## System Adaptation

Many of the rules in this manual are arbitrary in part and reflect a consensus of medical opinion rather than the result of controlled clinical trials. As medical opinion inevitably varies, so will the consensus of opinion about the proper rules for triage. This system can and should be modified to meet the needs of different settings; the only immutable requirement is that the rules be understood and agreed upon by all concerned. The following criteria should be observed in making changes: (1) changes must be made in writing; (2) changes must be made directly in the manual; (3) all persons affected by the change must be advised of that change before it is implemented. Verbal and spur-of-the-moment changes are inevitably a source of misunderstanding and confusion.

Adaptation based on a difference between the actual and assumed setting with respect to the providers of medical care available is considerably more straightforward than that necessitated by differences in medical opinion. For instance, if the family practitioner is replaced or augmented by an internist and a pediatrician, a very satisfactory adjustment is to simply add a rule whereby all patients under the age of thirteen referred to an M.D. are sent to the pediatrician and the rest are sent to the internist. Should an obstetrician-gynecologist be available, then the dispositions to "M.D." under gynecology may be changed to "OB-GYN."

In many cases it will be advantageous to triage by telephone. This necessitates changes to those rules dealing with individual complaints which assume the patient to be present. If these changes are to be made, it is necessary to rely on the triage worker to judge whether or not the patient has emergency signs. The possibility of an error in overestimating the severity of the problem must be accepted. If there is any suggestion of an emergency it is proper to ask the patient over the telephone if there is bleeding, shortness of breath, etc., but the triage worker must be willing to advise a STAT procedure if he or she cannot determine beyond a reasonable doubt that an emergency does not exist. Finally a practical definition of the STAT procedure must be devised. This could mean calling an ambulance, going to the nearest emergency room, coming immediately to the doctor's office or any other procedure deemed reasonable.

The author would appreciate greatly information on any adaptation of the system which is implemented. Indeed, any comment by those who use or attempt to use the system in any way would be most welcome.

# THE TRIAGE ENCOUNTER

## The First Concern

The first and foremost consideration with each patient is to determine whether or not that patient could be an emergency. The triage worker must learn to observe as well as to question the patient. If observation indicates that the patient needs immediate attention, then he should be sent directly to the physician without following any flowsheet.

Though everyone has decided at one time or another that someone *looked* sick, here are some things the triage worker should look for specifically:

1. Severe pain, as evidenced by complaint or action
2. Active bleeding
3. Stupor or drowsiness
4. Disorientation
5. Emotional disturbance
6. Dyspnea (shortness of breath) at rest
7. Cyanosis (blue color to lips, skin, or fingernails)
8. Extreme diaphoresis (profuse sweating—not related to environmental temperature)

These things must be considered with each patient. As the triage worker becomes more experienced, this will require little, if any, conscious effort. However, a feeling that the patient is quite ill should not be ignored because he does not have one of these symptoms. If there is any doubt, the physician must be consulted. On the other hand, it should *never* be assumed that the patient is *not* an emergency simply because he "looks all right." If nothing abnormal is revealed by observation of the patient, then the interview may begin.

## Patient Interview Techniques

The flowsheets will guide decision making. The techniques used to gather the data specified by the flowsheets are best learned during on-the-job training. The object is to gather data within the framework of a conversation so that the patient understands the questions, is put at ease, and feels that the triage worker is concerned about his problem. Some principles of patient interviewing are the following.

*Avoid leading questions.* In general, one should avoid asking questions in ways that lead the patient into giving answers he thinks are desired. This usually happens when the question is allowed to be answered with a simple "yes" or "no" when the question really is not simple and may have confused the patient. For example, if asked, "Do you have chest pain which is sharp and hurts more with coughing or deep breathing?" the patient may give a "yes" answer because he only heard "cough" or "pain" or simply because he thinks this must be an important question and does not want his problem underestimated. Preferably, the information should be obtained by asking less directive questions such as, "Do you have any pain?" and "What makes it worse?" There may be problems with being less direct in questioning, but as a rule the interview should at least begin in this manner.

*Keep the patient from rambling on.* Some patients will give long answers to relatively simple questions. The patient may seize upon a nondirect question as an opportunity for a half-hour chat. When confronted with such a patient, certain adjustments should be made in the interview technique. First, the patient should be interrupted when he or she begins to turn away from the subject of the question. This is best accomplished by asking another question or rephrasing the original question. Second, the questions may be made slightly more direct. Putting these two changes together, a fairly effective technique is to ask a series of short, simple questions to obtain the information. For example, if after asking about pain, the patient starts to talk about "a funny pain about six or seven years ago," one may interrupt with, "Do you have pain *now*?" When asked about the location of the pain, if the patient's response is vague, such as "all over" or "It's hard to say," the questions will have to be more specific. When becoming more specific, another useful technique is to offer a series of alternatives such as, "Is the pain in your legs or your belly or your chest or your arms?" rather than "Is the pain in your chest?" This may help to avoid the patient identifying a response that he thinks he should make because it sounds important.

### The Chief Complaint

The flowsheets start with only one complaint. However, the patient often has several complaints. Ideally, one would like to start with that complaint which eventually will be the most important medically. Determining which of the complaints fits this requirement is difficult or impossible to do at the beginning of the interview. A useful technique is to start with the complaint most important to the patient, that is, his *chief* complaint. This is determined simply by asking which complaint is most important or most troublesome to the patient.

As a rule, a diagnosis should not be accepted as a complaint. What the patient calls "indigestion" may be a heart attack. If a diagnosis is given as the chief complaint, the patient should be asked what symptoms suggested that diagnosis.

### Associated Complaints

After going through the flowsheet for a patient's chief complaint, the triage worker must determine if there are complaints not covered by that flowsheet. If there are complaints that have not been dealt with, then it must be determined whether or not another flowsheet must be used to triage those complaints. This determination can be made by looking at the associated complaints list at the bottom of many flowsheets. If the patient's non-triaged complaints are listed there, they need not be triaged, *provided* they *truly are associated* with the primary complaint. It usually is easy to tell that complaints are associated when they appear at the same time or during the same illness. If there is uncertainty about this, then each complaint should be triaged separately. If any complaint is *not* listed at the bottom of the sequence (even if it is associated with the primary complaint), then that complaint must be triaged using the appropriate flowsheet.

### Determining the Disposition of a Patient Triaged for Two or More Complaints

If a patient is triaged for more than one complaint, then more than one disposition may be indicated by the flowsheets. If this happens, disposition should be made according to the patient's highest priority complaint as determined by the list below. If the physician or physician's assistant is seen on a Today or STAT basis, he may elect to have the patient keep an appointment as suggested by triage.

Disposition priorities:
1. M.D. STAT
2. M.D.
3. P.A.
4. M.D. Appointments
5. Specialty Appointments

Children under three years are not seen by the physician's assistant; they should be referred directly to the physician.

### Vital Signs

The appropriate vital signs to be obtained are determined as a part of the triage process. These are listed at the bottom of the triage flowsheets. Vital signs are not obtained if the patient is sent to the M.D. STAT or if the patient is less than one year old. There are certain limits placed on these vital signs. If any of the measurements fall outside of these limits, it means that this measurement is abnormal to the point that a physician should see the patient promptly.

The limits are:

|  | Adults | 5-12 Years | 1-5 Years |
|---|---|---|---|
| BP: | Diastolic <60mmHg or >105mmHg | <60 or >85 | <50 or >75 |
|  | Systolic <90mmHg or >180mmHg | <90 or >150 | <70 or >120 |
| T: | >102° F | >102° F | >103° F |
| PULSE: | <50 or >120 or irregular | <60 or >120 | <80 or >150 |
| RR: | >28 | >36 | >44 |

## Ordering Laboratory Data

At the bottom of each flowsheet will be any laboratory data that is to be ordered. Be sure to include *STAT* if indicated on the flowsheet. Laboratory data ordered should be returned to the physician or physician's assistant who sees the patient.

## Writing the Problem-Oriented Note

A problem-oriented note consists of four sections: Subjective (history), Objective (physical, laboratory data, etc.), Assessment (diagnosis), and Plan. The acronym, SOAP, is sometimes used to indicate the four sections and their order.

A triage note usually has only Subjective and Plan sections because of the very brief encounter and lack of physical examination which characterize the triage process. An example of a triage note is included in the sample triage encounter.

## Sample Triage Encounter

A middle-aged woman patient, who is slightly obese, comes to be triaged. She is alert, moves without difficulty and has none of the symptoms for which the triage worker should look. Therefore, the triage worker concludes that she is in no distress and begins the interview.

"Good morning, I'm Mrs. Smith, and I'd like to ask a few questions in order to direct you to the most appropriate place for you to be seen today. First, can you tell me what is the *major* problem that led you to the clinic today?"

"Well, two days ago I began to have a strep throat and runny nose, and now I have a terrible headache that began last night and is just driving me crazy, and I have a corn on my foot and . . ."

At this point the triage worker has broken eye-to-eye contact and has begun to consult the triage manual. This has caused the patient to pause after a relatively short sentence. There are two immediate problems concerning what she has volunteered. First, she has given a diagnosis, "strep throat," for a complaint. While this probably translates rather reliably into "sore throat," it

should be asked what she means by strep throat. It is conceivable that she thinks she has a strep throat because of her having difficulty swallowing, swollen glands, etc. Second, the chief complaint must be determined so she is asked for the single complaint that bothers her most.

The patient confirms that by "strep throat" she means sore throat, and that this is her chief complaint.

Since the triage worker is not able to totally recall the sore throat flowsheet, she turns to it and asks the appropriate questions. The patient's answers (note that she has already answered the first and second questions in the flowsheet) indicate that she should be sent to the physician's assistant and that her temperature and pulse should be taken.

The patient's runny nose, which she clearly associates with her sore throat, is listed under Associated Complaints; therefore, it need not be considered further. The corn, however, has not been considered. The triage worker remembers this flowsheet so that she does not actually turn to it. When the patient states that her corn is not draining and only mildly annoying her, and the triage worker observes she is not limping, it is correctly concluded that a routine podiatrist appointment is appropriate. There are no vital signs indicated.

The physician's assistant disposition takes priority over the podiatrist appointment. The physician's assistant will decide if the patient should keep the appointment with the podiatrist. No laboratory tests are called for by the flowsheets.

The triage note might look something like this:

Name: Sanders, Mary          Date: 9/3/72

1.  Sore Throat

    Subjective—present for two days.

    Associated with headache.

    Objective—able to touch chin to chest.

    Plan—P.A. with temperature and pulse.

2. Corn

    Subjective—mildly annoying, not draining or causing a limp.

    Plan—Podiatrist Appointment, Routine.

Disposition: P.A.

Mary Smith

Note that the sore throat flowsheet is one of the few which asks for an objective piece of data, the ability to touch chin to chest.

## Overriding Disposition Rules, Triage Encounter

These are rules that supersede all others that might be found in this text.

### M.D. STAT

1. Any patient who appears severely ill.

2. Any patient whose vital signs are found to lie outside the prescribed limits.

### M.D.

Children less than three years old who are referred to the P.A. by flowsheets.

# HOW TO USE THIS MANUAL

By understanding the design of this manual, you should be able to find any complaint promptly.

On the following page is an index to flowsheets, listing twelve major clinical sections. Find the section in which you are interested and note that the page numbers for that section are aligned horizontally with the section title along the right-hand edge of the page. Turn to the index for your section. There the patient's individual complaints are listed.

All information pertaining to a complaint occupies only one page. The text appears on the left side of the page and is keyed numerically to the question rectangles in the corresponding flowsheet.

You should become familiar with the following abbreviations that are used in the flowsheets throughout this manual.

 An appointment should be made for the patient to see a doctor as soon as possible, usually within seven days of making that appointment.

The patient should be directed to a physician the same day the complaint is made.

 The patient has a possible emergent condition and should be directed to a physician immediately.

The patient's complaint can be handled by the physician's assistant as a routine matter.

The vital signs (VS) indicated below should be checked whenever the abbreviations appear on a flowsheet being followed. This may be the function of a nurse's aide or another person involved in the patient triage system.

BP—Blood Pressure

P—Pulse

RR—Respiratory Rate

T—Temperature

# GENERAL

# NEUROPSYCHIATRIC

# EYE

# EAR • NOSE • THROAT

# CARDIORESPIRATORY

# GASTROINTESTINAL

# GENITOURINARY

# GYNECOLOGICAL AND BREAST

# MUSCULO-SKELETAL

# PODIATRY

# DERMATOLOGY

# INDEX OF
# FLOWSHEETS

# MISCELLANEOUS

# GENERAL

## COMPLAINTS

# TRAUMA

This flowsheet will be useful only in instances of *minor* trauma since a patient with *major* trauma will be assumed to have one of the emergency signs.

1. This question simply reminds the triage worker to look for the emergency signs. Note that all patients with trauma go to the treatment room, regardless of who is to see the patient.

2. This is a list of the problems that the P.A. is able to investigate, and, in some cases, treat. Even if the problem is one requiring the attention of a physician, such as a facial laceration, the P.A. may perform the initial work-up and preparation of the patient. It is necessary to make a clear distinction between the traumas that can be treated only by an M.D. and those that can be treated by a P.A. (Flowsheets for this purpose are available.)

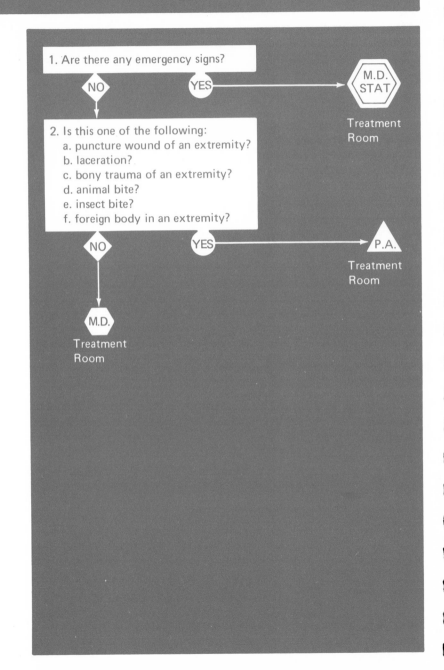

# FATIGUE

Fatigue may be associated with a wide variety of acute and chronic diseases. If there are any other symptoms present, triage is to be done on the basis of those symptoms. An exception is made in the case of a fever, since it is a relatively nonspecific symptom. Use of the fever flowsheet might lead to a circular process, since that flowsheet also directs the triage worker to associated symptoms, which possibly could be fatigue.

The most common cause of an isolated complaint of fatigue is emotional distress. However, the possibility of undiscovered illness remains. All in all, the complaint of fatigue alone requires the evaluation of an M.D.

Fever and chills are usually associated with an acute illness with other obvious symptoms. The triage workers must be sure to ask specifically about headache, rash, dysuria, sore throat, and cough, and vital signs must be checked before determining who the patient with isolated fever and chills will see. An exception is made of fatigue as an associated symptom since it is also rather nonspecific.

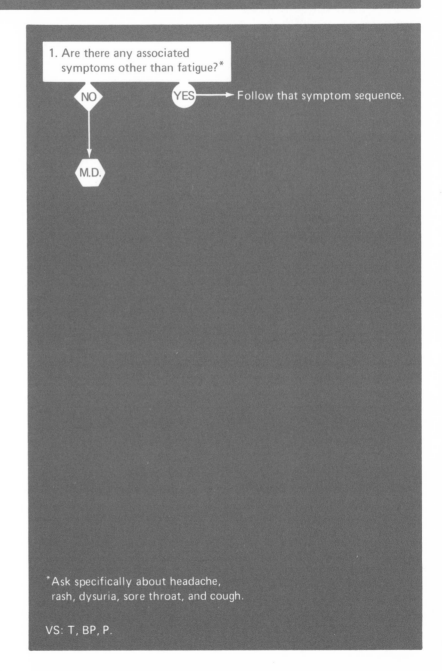

1. Are there any associated symptoms other than fatigue?*

NO

YES → Follow that symptom sequence.

M.D.

*Ask specifically about headache, rash, dysuria, sore throat, and cough.

VS: T, BP, P.

## SWOLLEN GLANDS

1. Most patients with the complaint of swollen glands have enlarged lymph nodes as a normal response to a viral illness. They should be triaged by their associated symptoms.

2. If the patient has recovered recently from a respiratory illness, he may be sent to the P.A. for evaluation. If this is an isolated complaint, or associated only with other constitutional symptoms, he should be seen by the M.D.

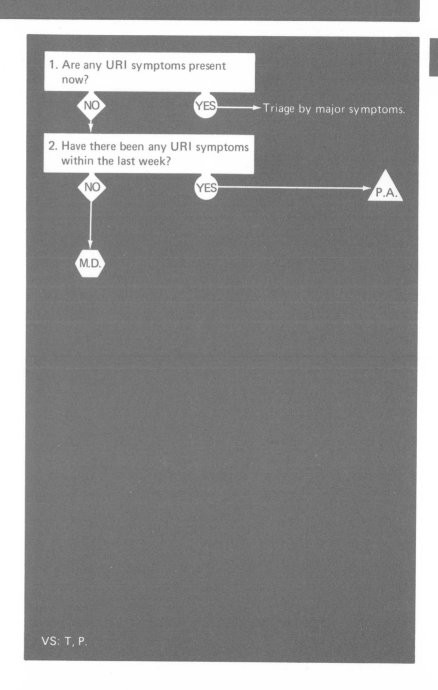

1. Are any URI symptoms present now?

NO

YES → Triage by major symptoms.

2. Have there been any URI symptoms within the last week?

NO

YES → P.A.

M.D.

VS: T, P.

**M.D.**

1. Any trauma not sent to the P.A.

2. Isolated fatigue, any patient.

3. Isolated fever and chills. (VS: T, BP, P.)

4. Swollen glands without current or recent (one week) symptoms of upper respiratory infection.

**P.A.**

1. Swollen glands associated with recent (one week) symptoms of upper respiratory infection. (VS: T, P.)

2. Trauma in the following categories:

   a. puncture wound of an extremity.
   b. laceration.
   c. bony trauma of an extremity.
   d. animal bite.
   e. insect bite.
   f. foreign body in an extremity.

# NEUROPSYCHIATRIC

## COMPLAINTS

Drowsiness and confusion often appear together and are not easily separated. Drowsiness means the patient is not alert; he appears sleepy. Confusion means he has trouble understanding simple questions. His attention span is short and his responses are inappropriate. It is possible to observe these symptoms even when the patient is relating other complaints.

1. Any change in alertness associated with recent head injury is a potentially unstable situation and requires an emergency disposition.

2. If the patient's drowsiness or confusion does not interfere significantly with his ability to relate a history, then it is mild.

3. Mild drowsiness or confusion is hard to distinguish from the fatigue or malaise that accompanies many acute and chronic illnesses. The patient's other complaints should be triaged, but a disposition to some care provider must be made for today. If this is the patient's only expressed problem, he should be seen by the M.D.

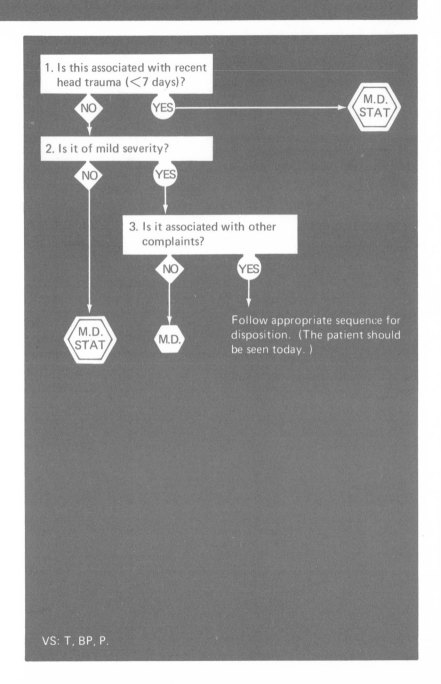

Often the patient will refer to his problem as "nerves" or as being upset, or he may use one of the words in the title above. The key is that the patient identifies the problem as one of mood, i.e., he doesn't feel good, but it is not because of a physical problem. These symptoms may be observed even if they are not mentioned by the patient.

1. A "yes" answer means that the patient does recognize the problem and is seeking help for such symptoms.

2. If the problem is a disturbance of mood, particularly extreme agitation, and it is severe enough to interfere with the triage worker's ability to obtain a triage history, then the patient should be referred to the M.D. On the other hand, a mild mood disturbance that is not recognized by the patient as a problem and does not interfere with the triage function requires only concerned care and interest in the patient. Some anxiety over medical problems is to be expected. The triage worker should take advantage of personal contact with the patient to help relieve the anxieties that often accompany other problems.

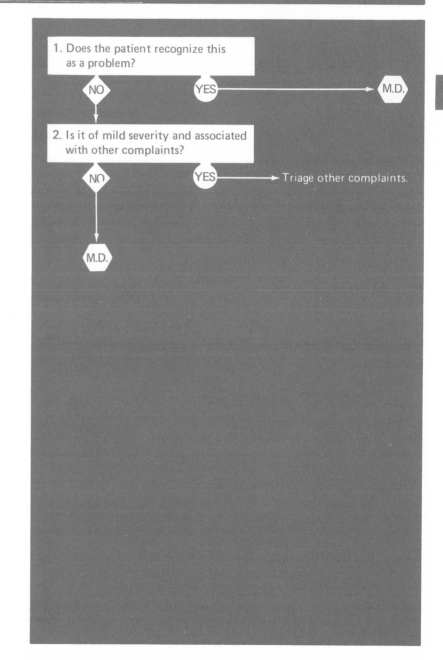

**9**

The terms *paralysis* and *weakness* refer to a loss of muscular strength. A complete loss is paralysis while a partial loss represents weakness.

1. The patient who complains of being "weak all over" is describing a manifestation of fatigue. Of more concern is the loss of muscular strength that is confined to one area of the body, commonly an arm, leg, or one side of the face.

2. A transient episode that is no longer giving the patient a problem needs to be evaluated today, but it is not an emergency.

3. A focal neurological deficit that is persistent or progressive and that has recently become a problem is a potentially unstable condition and requires an emergency evaluation.

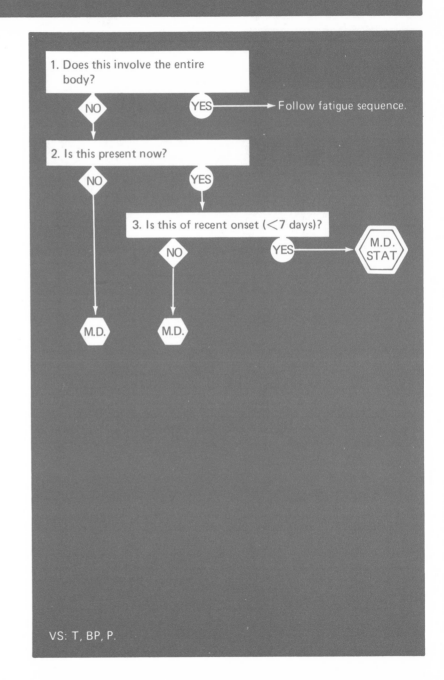

Any abnormal sensation in the skin surface is often described as numbness and occasionally as tingling or "pins and needles."

1. Numbness or tingling "all over the body" is not likely to be of neurological origin.

2. Abnormal sensations not associated with loss of muscle strength cannot adequately be triaged without objective data, which requires that an M.D. see the patient.

3. Persistent or progressive symptoms, including muscular weakness as well as sensory changes, need full evaluation by an M.D. The patient should be seen without delay if this is of recent onset.

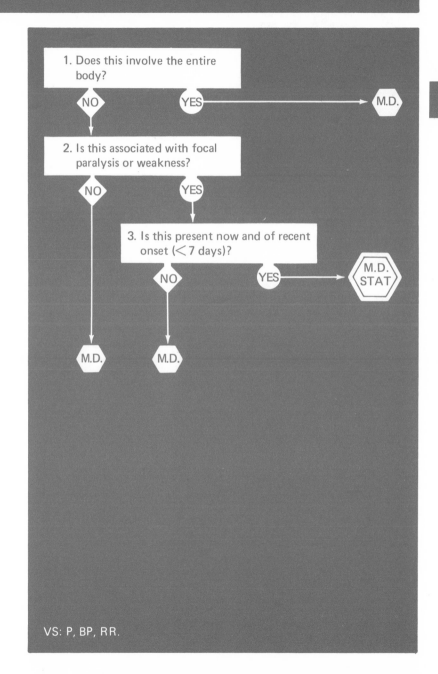

11

1. Does this involve the entire body?

NO · YES → M.D.

2. Is this associated with focal paralysis or weakness?

NO · YES

3. Is this present now and of recent onset (< 7 days)?

NO · YES → M.D. STAT

M.D. · M.D.

VS: P, BP, RR.

1. Any symptoms of altered mental function associated with recent head injury require emergency evaluation.

2. It is important to determine whether or not the patient has completely lost consciousness, regardless of cause. A patient who says he "almost fainted" or "may have blacked out for a few moments" has not completely lost consciousness. Refer the patient to an M.D. if you are uncertain.

3. A patient who has suffered a complete loss of consciousness usually arrives for medical evaluation promptly, and he requires emergency care. Those patients who, for some reason, wait more than twenty-four hours before seeking medical attention should be seen by an M.D. but not on an emergency basis.

4. If the patient says he is "dizzy," it is important to know exactly what he means by this. If he means "everything is spinning around" or "the floor seems to be moving," then he has vertigo. This is the type of dizziness that is produced, for example, by sea sickness or revolving on a merry-go-round. It is often accompanied by nausea, and, in children, it may present a staggering gait or loss of coordination.

5. Severe vertigo requires emergency disposition, primarily for the patient's comfort.

6. The other common type of dizziness is a lightheaded feeling. This often is described as faintness, a feeling that one is going to faint but doesn't actually lose consciousness. The patient's surroundings do not spin about, but they may seem to fade away or recede into the distance. It may come about by quickly standing or sitting up (postural hypotension). If the triage worker is unsure of what the patient means by "dizziness," an M.D. should see the patient.

7. A mild degree of faintness is a common manifestation of the malaise that frequently accompanies an illness. If this is the case, then triage the patient's major complaint to arrive at a disposition. If the patient complains of faintness as his major problem, then he should be seen by an M.D., even if there are associated, but less severe, symptoms.

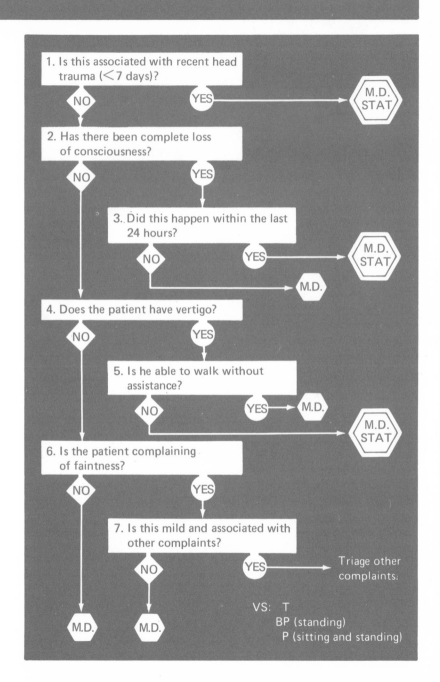

# HEADACHE

One especially must be concerned about meningitis in patients who complain of headaches. With any patient under thirty years old, the first concern must be that of not missing a case of meningitis. The triage worker should not hesitate to consult an M.D. if the patient in this age group does not appear alert and well.

1. By asking this question the triage worker hopes to detect meningismus, an important sign of meningitis. You simply ask the patient to touch his chin to his chest. With meningismus, the patient would be unable to do this because of spasms in the neck muscles.

2. Headache associated with recent trauma is a potentially unstable situation and requires an emergency disposition.

3. Children must be treated more conservatively than adults because headache is an unusual pediatric complaint, and early meningitis may be difficult to recognize in children.

4. The P.A. should not see a patient with the complaint of a headache without consulting an M.D. unless it is part of an upper respiratory infection symptom complex. The isolated complaint of a headache may be difficult to investigate, and the eventual diagnosis may rest on the interpretation of subtle clinical information.

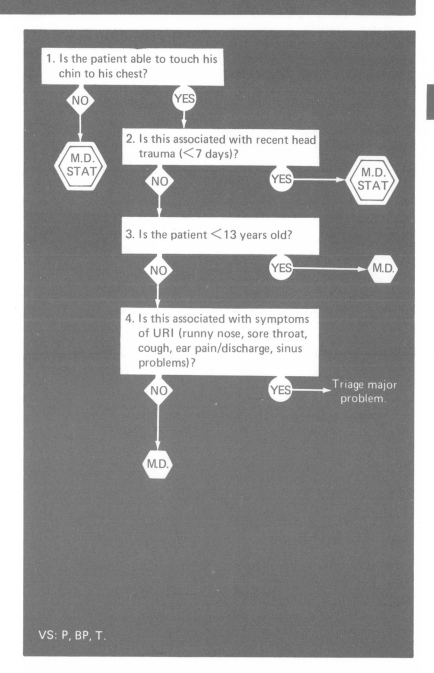

## M.D. STAT

1. Any of the following associated with recent (less than seven days) trauma:

   a. drowsiness and/or confusion.
   b. dizziness, faintness, or blackout.
   c. headache.

2. Severe drowsiness and/or confusion.

3. Complete loss of consciousness within the last twenty-four hours.

4. Adult patient with symptoms of drowsiness and/or confusion that is more than mildly severe.

5. Paralysis and/or weakness that is:

   a. focal.
   b. persistent.
   c. of recent (less than seven days) onset.

6. Vertigo, patient unable to walk without assistance.

7. Headache, patient unable to touch his chin to his chest.

## M.D.

1. Mild drowsiness and/or confusion without other symptoms.

2. Any patient showing symptoms of depression, nervousness, anxiety, or tension that are more than mildly severe.

3. Numbness and/or tingling involving the total body and/or not associated with focal paralysis or weakness.

4. Complete loss of consciousness that:

   a. is not associated with recent head trauma.
   b. occurred more than twenty-four hours ago.

5. Dizziness that:

   a. is not associated with recent head trauma.
   b. did not cause loss of consciousness.
   c. cannot be defined as either vertigo or faintness.

6. Faintness that:

   a. is not associated with recent head injury.
   b. did not cause loss of consciousness.
   c. is the patient's chief complaint.

7. Focal paralysis and weakness that is:

   a. transient (not present now).
   b. chronic (more than seven days).
   (VS: T, P, BP. Also RR if associated with numbness or tingling.)

8. Vertigo, patient able to walk without assistance.
   (VS: P (sitting and standing), BP (standing), T.)

9. Headache that:

   a. is not associated with URI symptoms.
   b. is not associated with recent head trauma.
   c. is associated with ability to touch chin to chest.
   (VS: BP, P, T.)

10. Headache in a patient who is less than thirteen years old.

# EYE

## COMPLAINTS

# EYE INJURY

Any injury or trauma to the eye including those which may have left a foreign body in the eye. The foreign body flowsheet is intended for use when the foreign body is not associated with a blow or other trauma.

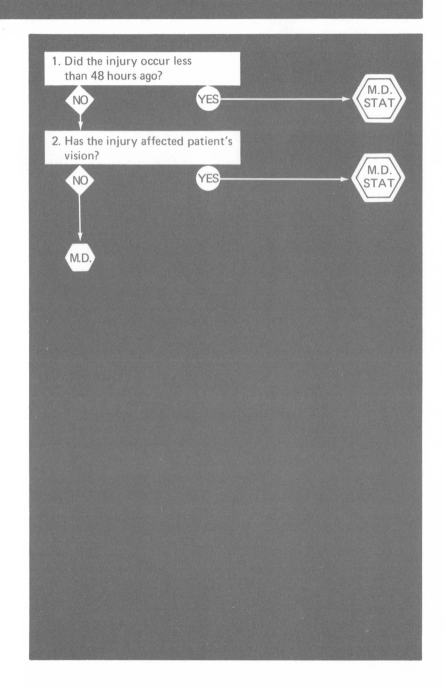

1. Did the injury occur less than 48 hours ago?

NO     YES → M.D. STAT

2. Has the injury affected patient's vision?

NO     YES → M.D. STAT

NO → M.D.

Pain includes burning sensations. Discharge often causes crusting on the eyelids, especially in the morning.

1. For reasons of patient comfort, as well as possible serious problems, patients with more than mild discomfort will be sent to the M.D.

2. Certain cases of conjunctivitis may be treated by a P.A. The presence of any other eye symptoms make uncomplicated conjunctivitis questionable, and these patients should be handled in a different manner.

17

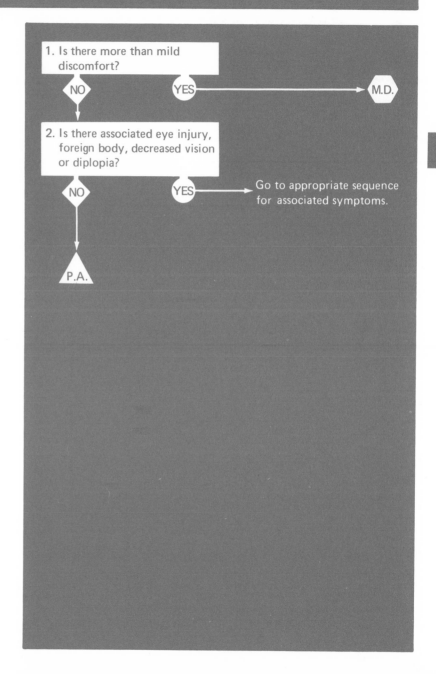

1. Is there more than mild discomfort?

NO    YES ──────────────→ M.D.

2. Is there associated eye injury, foreign body, decreased vision or diplopia?

NO    YES ──────→ Go to appropriate sequence for associated symptoms.

P.A.

## FOREIGN BODY IN EYE

The patient does not need to be positive that something is in his eye. Most of us feel a specific sensation when a foreign body is present in the eye, so if the patient thinks it is a foreign body, then his word is sufficient. If there is any question that there could be a foreign body imbedded in the eye, then the eye should be examined without delay.

18

Images are less distinct or a portion of the visual field is now "blacked out" with decreased vision.

1. All of the symptoms listed here may signify serious problems and deserve the immediate attention of the M.D. The triage worker should be conservative. Always ask the M.D. if you are not sure. If none of these symptoms are present, then the P.A. may test visual acuity and visual fields before referring the patient to the M.D.

19

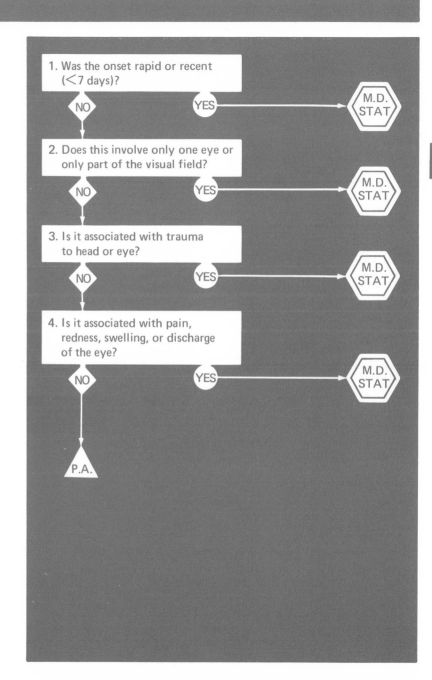

# DIPLOPIA

Diplopia means seeing double images. This complaint may be difficult to evaluate so it should be sent to the M.D.

# SEEING SPOTS

The patient may state that he sees "stars," "flashes," or "floaters."

1 and 2.   Sudden onset and/or loss of either a portion of the visual field or blurring of vision may indicate a detached retina. If the symptoms are not present, a P.A. may evaluate their visual acuity and visual fields before consulting an M.D. The common "floaters" are usually associated with myopia (nearsightedness).

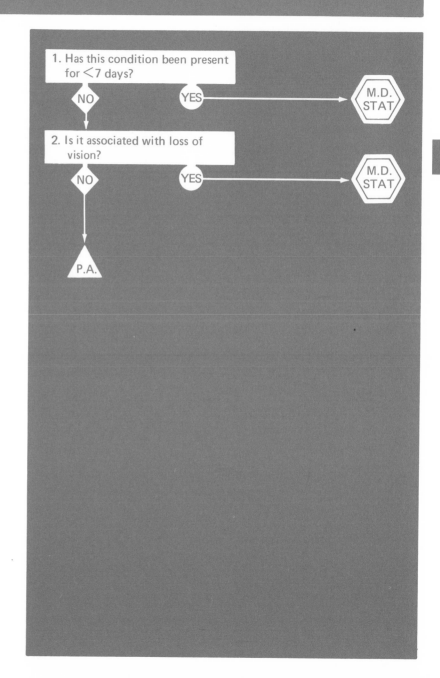

## GLASSES REQUEST

This should be considered a request for a service and must be distinguished from serious problems that the patient hopes to solve with glasses. The most common problem that leads to such a request is decreased vision. Seeing spots, eye pain, and headache are others. Such problems must be recognized and triaged by their respective flowsheets. The patient should be sent directly to a P.A. only when it is certain that glasses are all that is required.

# EYELID PROBLEM

By far the most common complaint in this group will be that of a "stye." The triage worker should be sure that the problem is confined to the eyelid and it is not part of a generalized condition.

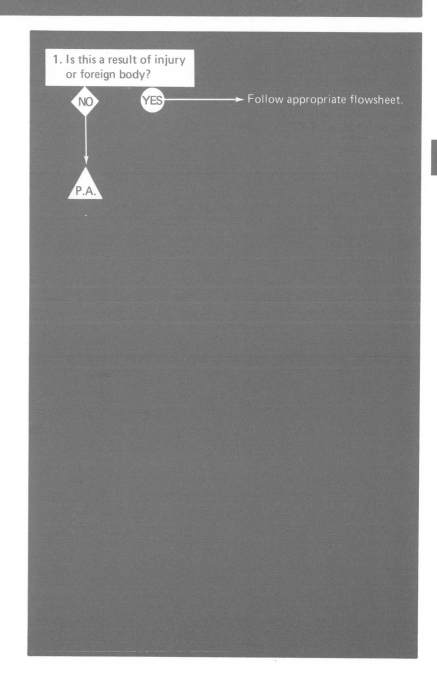

1. Is this a result of injury or foreign body?

NO

YES → Follow appropriate flowsheet.

P.A.

## M.D. STAT

1. Any eye injury within the last forty-eight hours.

2. Foreign body sensation in the eye.

3. Decreased vision with any of the following:

   a. rapid or recent onset (less than seven days).
   b. only one eye or only part of the visual field.
   c. trauma to head or eye.
   d. pain, redness, swelling, or discharge.

4. Seeing spots, with either:

   a. recent onset (less than seven days).
   b. loss of vision.

## M.D.

1. Any eye injury more than forty-eight hours old.

2. Any eye pain, irritation or discharge with more than mild discomfort.

3. Any patient with diplopia.

## P.A.

1. Eye pain and/or itching, and/or discharge with mild discomfort and *none* of the following:

   a. eye injury.
   b. foreign body sensation.
   c. decreased vision.
   d. diplopia.

2. Eyelid problem not associated with injury or foreign body.

3. Seeing spots and condition is:

   a. chronic (more than seven days).
   b. not associated with loss of vision.

4. Request for glasses, no eye symptoms.

5. Decreased vision that:

   a. is slow in onset (more than seven days).
   b. involves both eyes and entire visual field.
   c. is not associated with head or eye trauma.
   d. is not associated with eye pain, redness, swelling or discharge.

## EAR • NOSE • THROAT

### COMPLAINTS

When a child is observed tugging or pulling at his ear, it is possible that one or more of the above problems exist. The triage worker should always ask about the possibility of a foreign body, particularly in children, and if a foreign body is present, the appropriate sequence should be followed.

1. Ear infections can be complicated by meningitis, so the triage worker should always ask about headaches.

2. Headache with meningismus will be evaluated promptly by an M.D. Associated headache without meningismus is common and nonspecific. It will be evaluated by a P.A.

3 and 4.  Chronic symptoms or associated vertigo suggest more complicated or serious problems, and the patient should be seen by an M.D.

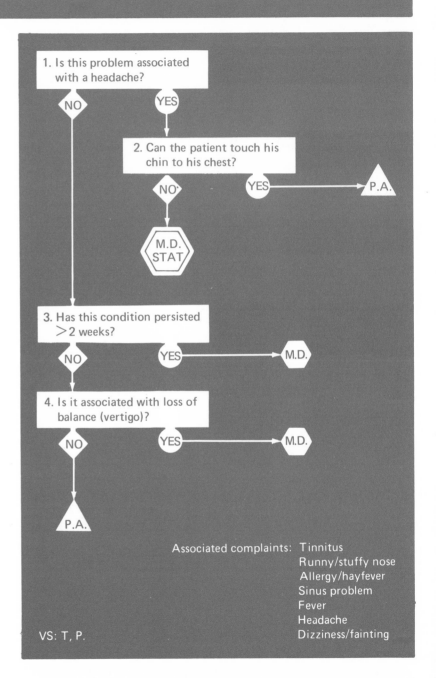

1. Is this problem associated with a headache?
NO — YES
2. Can the patient touch his chin to his chest?
NO — YES → P.A.
M.D. STAT
3. Has this condition persisted >2 weeks?
NO — YES → M.D.
4. Is it associated with loss of balance (vertigo)?
NO — YES → M.D.
P.A.

VS: T, P.

Associated complaints:  Tinnitus
Runny/stuffy nose
Allergy/hayfever
Sinus problem
Fever
Headache
Dizziness/fainting

# TINNITUS

Tinnitus is a ringing in the ears.

1. Vertigo or "room-spinning dizziness" is a symptom of inner ear problems. It is often associated with nausea. In children, the triage worker should ask about loss of balance, frequent falling down or wandering into walls. This should be distinguished from lightheadedness, a frequent complaint with viral infections.

2. Severe vertigo is triaged to an M.D. STAT, primarily for the patient's comfort.

3. Fluid in the middle ear, wax in the canal, perforations of the tympanic membrane, and otitis media are probably the most common causes of tinnitus. The P.A.'s rule for tinnitus will exclude the occasional patient with another cause who also has an upper respiratory infection.

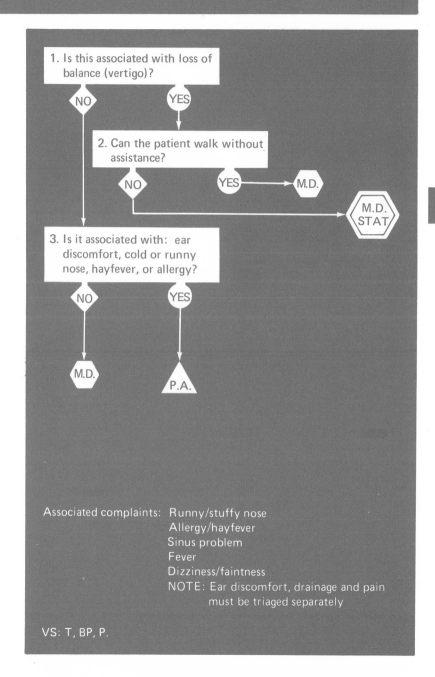

1. Is this associated with loss of balance (vertigo)?
   - NO
   - YES

2. Can the patient walk without assistance?
   - NO
   - YES → M.D.

M.D. STAT

3. Is it associated with: ear discomfort, cold or runny nose, hayfever, or allergy?
   - NO → M.D.
   - YES → P.A.

Associated complaints:  Runny/stuffy nose
                        Allergy/hayfever
                        Sinus problem
                        Fever
                        Dizziness/faintness
                        NOTE: Ear discomfort, drainage and pain
                              must be triaged separately

VS: T, BP, P.

## FOREIGN BODY IN EAR OR NOSE

Adults will know if a foreign body is present. In children, the triage worker must ask if they had been playing with small objects or had been eating before the difficulty. Peas, corn, peanuts and beads are common objects.

M.D.
STAT

# OTHER HEARING PROBLEMS

Patients with nonspecific hearing problems will be interviewed and examined by a P.A. before seeing an M.D. Note that tinnitus (ringing in the ears) is triaged separately.

# WAX IN EAR

The triage worker should try to distinguish a true complaint of hearing loss (attributed by patient to wax in his ear) from bothersome wax. Both, however, will be seen by a P.A.

A runny or stuffy nose generally indicates a cold, although allergy, streptococcal infection (if patient is less than two years old), foreign body, and/or tumor may be the cause. The P.A. will evaluate the patient's symptoms. The triage worker should be sure to ask about foreign bodies and allergies.

P.A.

Associated complaints: Sinus problem
Fever
Allergy/hayfever
Muscle aches

VS: T.

This is a chief complaint which a P.A. will evaluate and then treat or refer the patient accordingly.

P.A.

Associated complaints: Runny/stuffy nose
Sinus problem
Fever ،
Muscle aches

VS: T.

# SINUS PROBLEM

The P.A. is responsible for further characterizing the problem as infectious, allergic, possible tumor, etc. If the problem is an acute infection, treatment will be given. Otherwise, the patient will be referred to an appropriate specialist by a P.A.

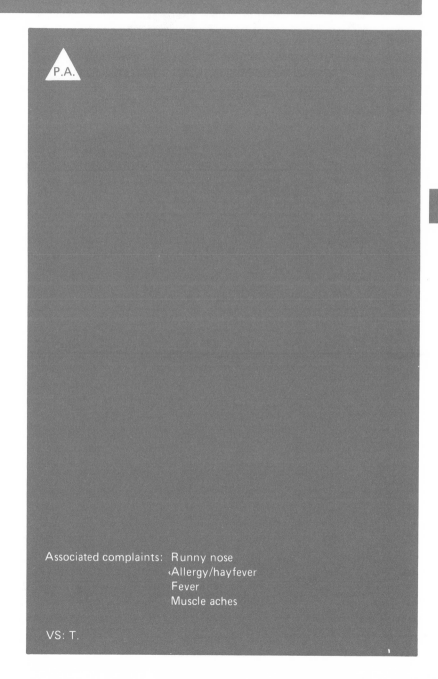

P.A.

Associated complaints:  Runny nose
                        ‹Allergy/hayfever
                        Fever
                        Muscle aches

VS: T.

# EPISTAXIS

This flowsheet is to be used for nose bleeds only. The triage worker must ask questions to distinguish this problem from coughing up blood or spitting up blood, conditions that originate in the mouth or stomach. Mild nosebleeds frequently are secondary to the nasal inflammation of a cold. The P.A. can evaluate and treat this.

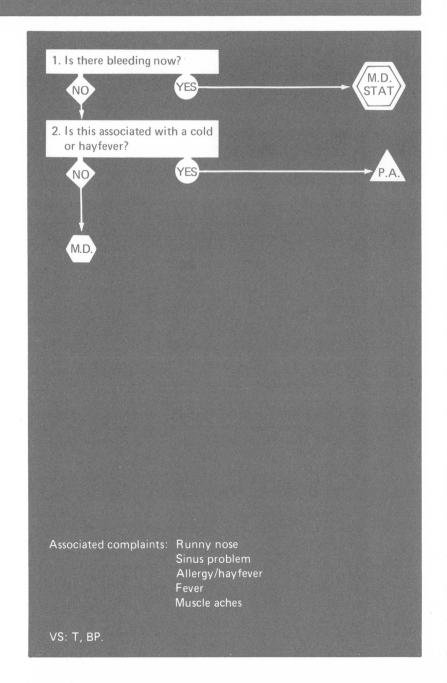

1. Is there bleeding now?

NO    YES ──────────────────► M.D. STAT

2. Is this associated with a cold or hayfever?

NO    YES ──────────────────► P.A.

M.D.

Associated complaints:  Runny nose
                        Sinus problem
                        Allergy/hayfever
                        Fever
                        Muscle aches

VS: T, BP.

# SORE THROAT

The common complaint of sore throat generally is caused by a viral infection. This is true in seventy percent or more of the cases. In order to treat bacterial infection and possible seriousness of late streptococcal complications, proper evaluation is important.

1. A chronic sore throat may be due to chronically infected tonsils, mononucleosis, or, occasionally, malignancy, and should be evaluated by an M.D.

2 and 3.  Sore throat can be the presenting complaint of meningitis. These two questions are now familiar as the method of screening for this complication in a triage setting.

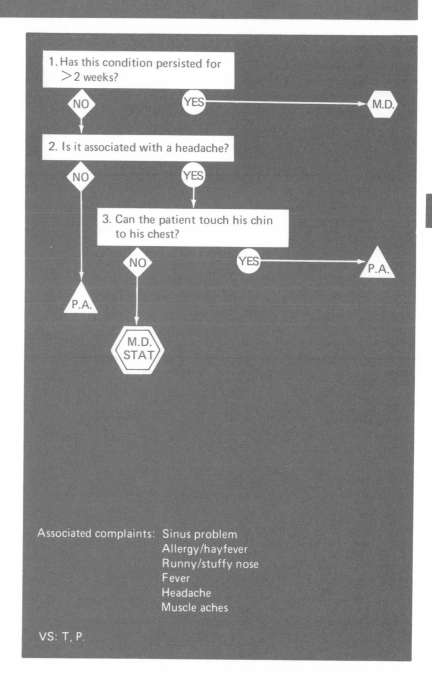

1. Has this condition persisted for >2 weeks?
   NO    YES → M.D.

2. Is it associated with a headache?
   NO    YES

3. Can the patient touch his chin to his chest?
   NO    YES → P.A.

P.A.

M.D. STAT

Associated complaints:  Sinus problem
                        Allergy/hayfever
                        Runny/stuffy nose
                        Fever
                        Headache
                        Muscle aches

VS: T, P.

1. This is a fairly common associated symptom during an active upper respiratory infection. Its presence does not alter the triage of other symptoms, even if hoarseness and laryngitis seem to be the major symptoms.

2. Hoarseness and laryngitis may persist after other URI symptoms have resolved. The P.A. will evaluate this situation. If this is an isolated complaint, however, the M.D. should see the patient.

36

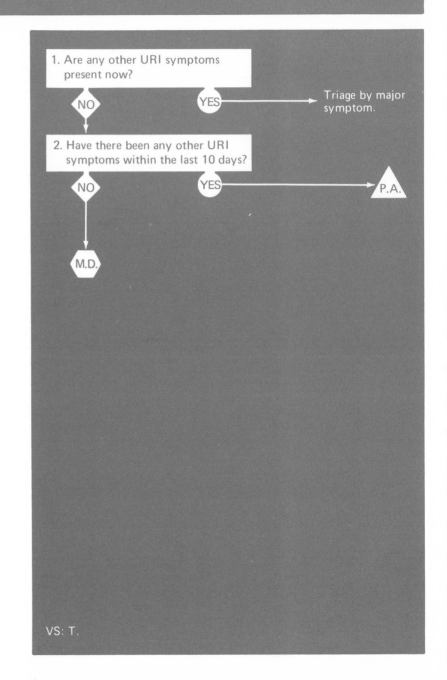

1. Are any other URI symptoms present now?

NO   YES → Triage by major symptom.

2. Have there been any other URI symptoms within the last 10 days?

NO   YES → P.A.

M.D.

VS: T.

**M.D. STAT**

1. Tinnitus with vertigo (patient unable to walk without assistance).

2. Active epistaxis.

3. Ear drainage, pain, and/or discomfort or sore throat with headache and patient unable to touch chin to chest.

**M.D.**

1. Isolated tinnitus (no vertigo or URI symptoms).

2. Ear drainage, pain, and/or discomfort that is either chronic (duration of more than two weeks) or associated with vertigo.

3. Nose or ear trauma more than forty-eight hours old.

4. Hoarseness and/or laryngitis not associated with recent (one week) or current URI symptoms.

5. Foreign body in ear or nose.

6. Tinnitus associated with mild to moderate vertigo (patient able to walk unassisted).
(VS: T, P, BP.)

7. Epistaxis that is not active and not associated with cold or hayfever.
(VS: BP, T.)

8. Chronic (more than two weeks) sore throat.
(VS: P, T.)

**P.A.**

1. Wax in ear.

2. Hearing problem.

3. Tinnitus without vertigo but associated with URI symptoms.
(VS: T, P, BP.)

4. Ear drainage, pain, and/or discomfort without vertigo and of recent onset (less than two weeks). May be associated with headache if patient able to touch chin to chest.
(VS: T, P.)

5. Runny or stuffy nose.
(VS: T.)

6. Allergy or hayfever.
(VS: T.)

7. Sinus problem.
(VS: T.)

8. Epistaxis that is not active but is associated with cold or hayfever.
(VS: T, BP.)

9. Sore throat of recent onset (less than two weeks).
(VS: T, P.)

10. Hoarseness and/or laryngitis associated with recent (one week) URI symptoms.
(VS: T.)

37

# CARDIORESPIRATORY

## COMPLAINTS

This flowsheet is to be used only when the sensation experienced by the patient is that of not getting enough air. "Air hunger" or "feelings of suffocation" are descriptive of this sensation. This symptom is *always* exacerbated by exertion. Indeed, it is the same sensation we all experience after strenuous activity.

Having trouble breathing is not the same as shortness of breath. It is important to understand what the patient means by trouble breathing. If it is because of a stuffy nose, chest pain, persistent cough, or generalized fatigue, then his complaint must be triaged by the appropriate sequence.

1. The patient who is truly short of breath at rest is in significant respiratory distress and should see the M.D. immediately. Such a situation usually is obvious in an adult. In an infant, the triage worker should observe carefully, as well as ask the parents, for such things as grunting respirations, flaring of the nostrils, and retraction (pulling in of the skin between and beneath the ribs with each breath). The triage worker should consult with the M.D. *immediately* if there is any doubt.

2. The cough–wheeze sequence will give an appropriate disposition, even when these symptoms are complicated by a mild to moderate degree of shortness of breath. Isolated shortness of breath is a complicated situation that requires evaluation by the M.D.

40

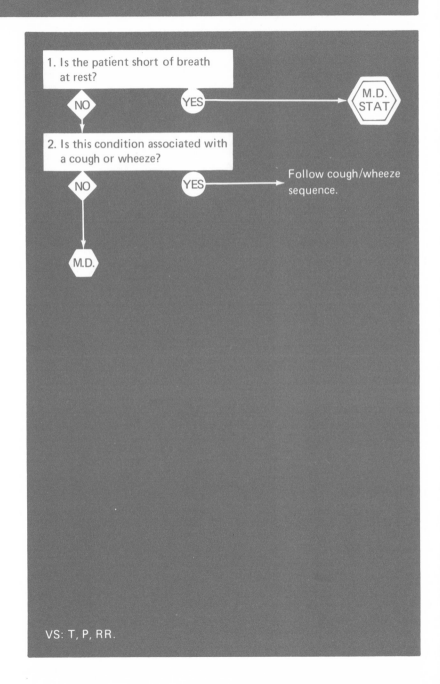

# CHEST PAIN

This means pain anywhere in the chest area; however, it needs to be distinguished from back pain and generalized muscle aches. When the patient's chief complaint is chest pain, the triage worker should be especially alert to his general appearance. As always, if the patient is in distress, he should see the M.D. promptly. A conservative approach must be used with this complaint, particularly in patients over thirty years old.

1. This question is discussed under shortness of breath sequence.

2. To be conservative, the triage worker should consult promptly with the M.D. if the patient is over thirty years old and is having more than mild pain in his chest.

3. Pain made worse by deep breathing is due to a sore chest wall or to pleurisy. Pain made worse by coughing may have the same significance but may also be a "searing" substernal pain that may occur in any patient with a prolonged or vigorous cough. A sore chest that is tender to the touch indicates the presence of a musculo-skeletal syndrome, as does pain that is exacerbated by twisting movements of the chest wall. Patients with pain which is not clearly described by any of the above should be seen promptly by the M.D.

4. The cough–wheeze flowsheet will lead to an appropriate disposition even if these symptoms are complicated by chest pain as described in question 3. In the absence of a cough, this type of chest pain is most likely to be a chest-wall syndrome, although there are still other possibilities (such as pericarditis). This can be initially evaluated by the P.A.

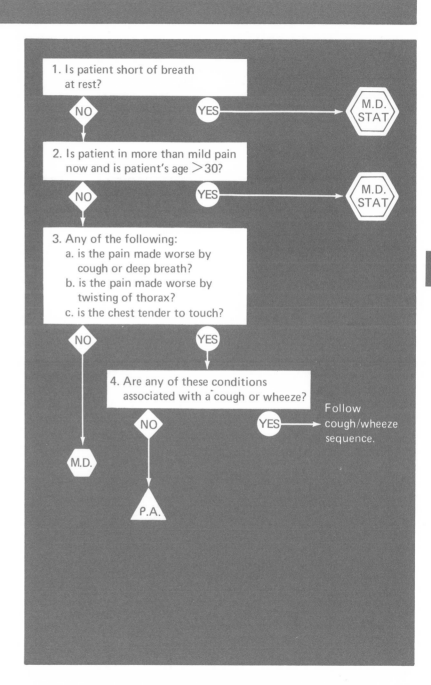

41

A cough should need no definition. A wheeze is a dry, "musical" whistling sound produced by air forced through narrowed passages. It is always more pronounced during expiration, and it often is completely absent during inspiration. Gurgling or bubbling respiratory noises are not wheezes. Common symptoms (such as headache, ear pain, chest pain, sore throat) which are *not* on the list of associated symptoms must be triaged separately if they are present.

1. This question is discussed under the shortness of breath sequence. It should also be noted that a patient who is wheezing during *inspiration* is likely to be in respiratory distress, i.e., to be short of breath at rest.

2. Rusty or blood-streaked sputum is *not* what is meant by grossly bloody sputum. A patient with the latter should be sent directly to the M.D. The triage worker should consult the M.D. if in doubt.

3. This means that wheezing is audible without the use of a stethoscope. The triage worker should determine whether or not the wheezing is due to a stuffy nose by having the patient breathe through his mouth.

4. A cough that is of recent onset is evaluated by the P.A. A chronic cough may require more extensive evaluation.

42

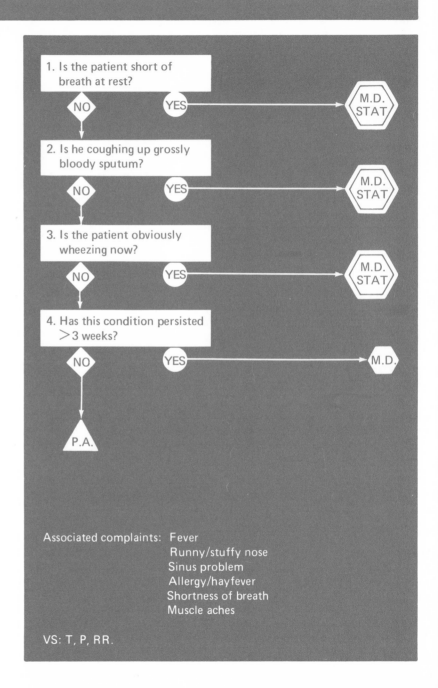

1. Is the patient short of breath at rest?
   NO / YES → M.D. STAT

2. Is he coughing up grossly bloody sputum?
   NO / YES → M.D. STAT

3. Is the patient obviously wheezing now?
   NO / YES → M.D. STAT

4. Has this condition persisted >3 weeks?
   NO / YES → M.D.

P.A.

Associated complaints: Fever
Runny/stuffy nose
Sinus problem
Allergy/hayfever
Shortness of breath
Muscle aches

VS: T, P, RR.

**M.D. STAT**

1. Patient short of breath at rest.

2. Presence of grossly bloody sputum.

3. Patient obviously wheezing now.

4. More than mild chest pain that is now present, and patient over thirty.

**M.D.**

1. Shortness of breath, not present at rest and not associated with a cough and/or a wheeze.

2. Chest pain that:

   a. is not made worse by cough, deep breathing or twisting of thorax.
   b. is not tender to touch.
   c. patient is not short of breath at rest.

3. Chronic cough or wheeze (more than three weeks duration) and:

   a. patient not short of breath at rest.
   b. patient not producing grossly bloody sputum.

c. patient not wheezing now.
   (VS: T, P, RR.)

4. Chest pain that:

   a. is associated with a cough and/or a wheeze as defined above.
   b. is made worse by coughing, deep breathing, twisting, or is tender to touch.
   (VS: T, P, RR.)

**P.A.**

1. Mild chest pain (made worse by coughing, deep breathing, twisting, or tender to touch) and:

   a. patient is not short of breath at rest.
   b. patient is under thirty years of age.
   c. not associated with a cough and/or a wheeze, or associated with a cough and/or a wheeze as defined below.
   (VS: T, P, BP.)

2. A cough and/or a wheeze of recent onset (less than three weeks) and:

   a. patient not short of breath at rest.
   b. no presence of grossly bloody sputum.
   c. patient not obviously wheezing at rest.
   (VS: T, P, RR.)

43

# GASTROINTESTINAL

## COMPLAINTS

These three symptoms are triaged together because they so frequently accompany one another in illness. In triaging any or all three symptoms, the flowsheets are to be used in exactly the same way. Nausea means a sickness to the stomach with an inclination to vomit. Diarrhea means loose or liquid bowel movements, usually more frequent than normal.

2. (A.)  Recent head injury is serious because bleeding inside the skull can cause increased pressure on the brain. This, associated with nausea and vomiting, can lead to a coma and the patient's death.

(B and C.)  Black or bloody vomitus or stools may represent serious internal gastrointestinal bleeding, requiring immediate transfusions of fluid and blood. The vomitus or stool turns black because of the action of gastric juices on hemoglobin, and usually represents bleeding from the esophagus, stomach or duodenum. Bloody vomitus may look like coffee grounds or it may be red if it is very fresh.

(D.)  Determining the severity of abdominal pain is a very subjective matter. Some patients tend to overreact; others tend to minimize the pain when they are asked about its severity. Any patient who appears visibly disturbed with pain, who is clutching his abdomen, or who is bent over should be referred to the M.D. STAT. On the other hand, the triage worker should accept the patient's estimation that the pain is severe even if the patient "looks well."

3. A missed or late period means pregnancy is possible.

4. By asking these questions, you attempt to differentiate more serious cases that should be triaged directly to the M.D.

5. Diabetics with nausea, vomiting, and/or diarrhea may be having serious complications of their disease. Likewise, those with more than eight stools in twenty-four hours may be significantly dehydrated.

Often, prescribed medications such as antibiotics or birth control pills may have side effects of nausea, vomiting, and/or diarrhea. The M.D. will have to decide if the symptoms may be due to side effects.

46

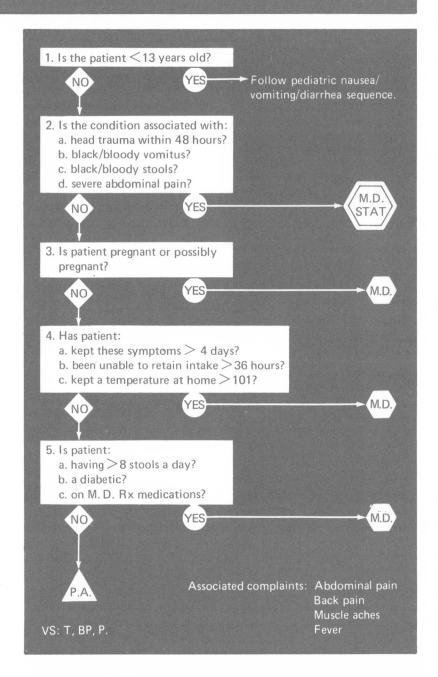

1. Is the patient < 13 years old?

NO    YES → Follow pediatric nausea/vomiting/diarrhea sequence.

2. Is the condition associated with:
   a. head trauma within 48 hours?
   b. black/bloody vomitus?
   c. black/bloody stools?
   d. severe abdominal pain?

NO    YES → M.D. STAT

3. Is patient pregnant or possibly pregnant?

NO    YES → M.D.

4. Has patient:
   a. kept these symptoms > 4 days?
   b. been unable to retain intake > 36 hours?
   c. kept a temperature at home > 101?

NO    YES → M.D.

5. Is patient:
   a. having > 8 stools a day?
   b. a diabetic?
   c. on M. D. Rx medications?

NO    YES → M.D.

P.A.

VS: T, BP, P.

Associated complaints: Abdominal pain
Back pain
Muscle aches
Fever

# PEDIATRIC NAUSEA • VOMITING • DIARRHEA

These three symptoms are triaged together because they frequently accompany one another. In triaging any or all of these symptoms, the flowsheets are to be used in exactly the same way. Nausea is a common complaint in children who are old enough to verbalize this problem. However, it often must be inferred from the actions of the young child who is unable to be specific about this type of problem. Diarrhea in infants must be judged by the number of stools as well as the consistency.

1. Although diarrhea in children is common, bloody stools may represent serious, communicable infections such as salmonella, shigella, or pathogenic E. coli, and the isolation room disposition is necessary.

2. (A.) Recent head injury is serious because bleeding inside the skull can cause increased pressure on the brain. This, associated with nausea and vomiting, can lead to a coma and the patient's death.

(B and C.) Black or bloody vomitus may represent serious upper gastrointestinal bleeding requiring immediate transfusions. The blood may look black or like coffee grounds because of the action of gastric juices. Most children will have some discomfort with nausea, vomiting, and/or diarrhea; however, if the child appears to be in extreme discomfort, e.g., clutching his abdomen or bent over, he should be sent to the M.D. STAT.

3. This question and the following question attempt to determine if the patient is having more severe episodes of nausea, vomiting, and/or diarrhea and should be referred directly to the M.D.

4. Diabetics with nausea, vomiting, and/or diarrhea may be having serious complications and should be seen immediately by the M.D. Frequently, prescribed medicines such as antibiotics may cause nausea, vomiting, and/or diarrhea. In these cases, the patient should be seen by the M.D.

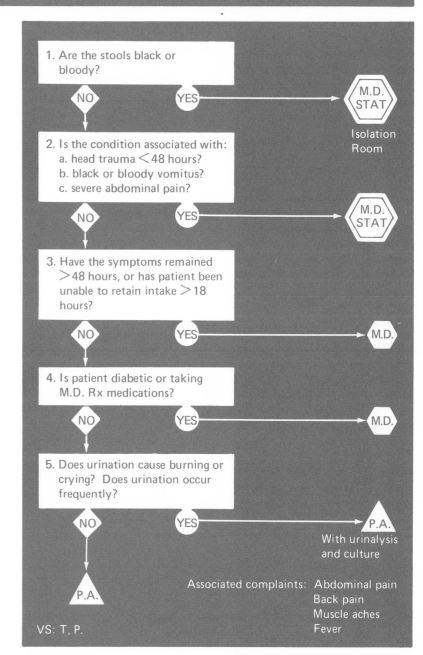

47

Abdominal pain is pain anywhere below the ribs and above the groin in the front half of the body. It may have literally hundreds of causes.

3. (A.) Black stools, that may resemble tar, may represent serious bleeding anywhere along the gastrointestinal tract.

(B.) A recent injury or blow to the abdomen could suggest an emergency situation, e.g., a ruptured spleen.

(C.) Determining the severity of abdominal pain is a very subjective matter. Some patients tend to overreact; others tend to minimize pain when asked about its severity. Any patient who appears visibly disturbed with pain, who is clutching his abdomen, or who is bent over, should be referred to the M.D. STAT. A patient who says his pain is severe also should be sent to the M.D. STAT.

4. A late or missed period is sufficient to send the patient to the M.D.

**48**

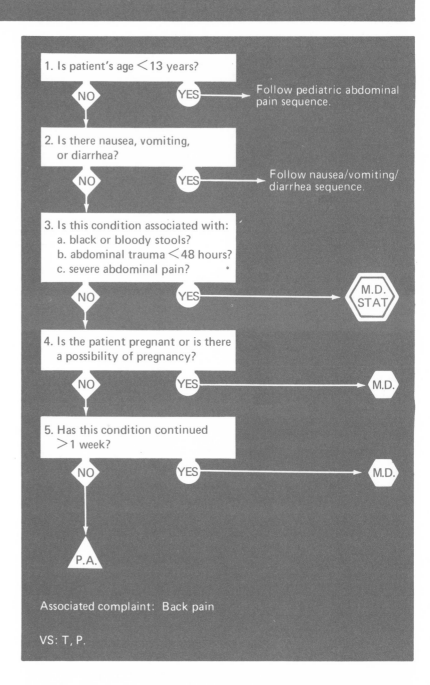

1. Is patient's age < 13 years?
 NO / YES → Follow pediatric abdominal pain sequence.

2. Is there nausea, vomiting, or diarrhea?
 NO / YES → Follow nausea/vomiting/diarrhea sequence.

3. Is this condition associated with:
 a. black or bloody stools?
 b. abdominal trauma < 48 hours?
 c. severe abdominal pain?
 NO / YES → M.D. STAT

4. Is the patient pregnant or is there a possibility of pregnancy?
 NO / YES → M.D.

5. Has this condition continued > 1 week?
 NO / YES → M.D.

P.A.

Associated complaint: Back pain

VS: T, P.

# PEDIATRIC ABDOMINAL PAIN

Abdominal pain is pain anywhere below the ribs and above the groin in the front half of the body. It may have literally hundreds of causes. In infants, abdominal pain must be inferred from their actions, such as constant crying, holding of the abdomen, crying whenever someone touches a part of the belly, etc.

2. A recent injury or blow to the abdomen could suggest an emergency situation, e.g., ruptured spleen.

3. Pain, less than seventy-two hours in duration, deserves prompt investigation by the M.D.

4. These are symptoms of urinary tract infection and other kidney/bladder problems; hence, they determine whether a urine specimen will be obtained.

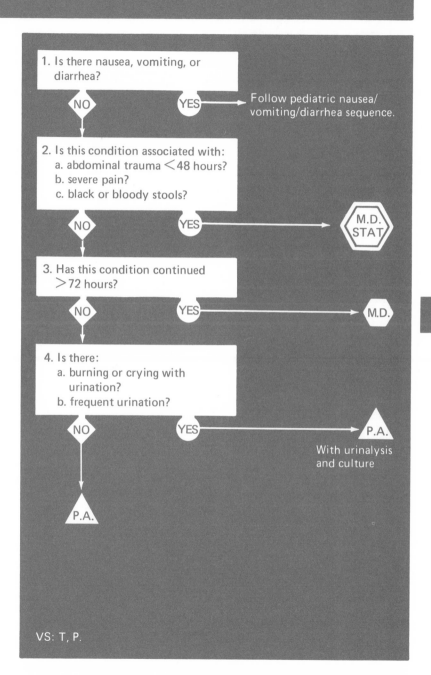

1. Is there nausea, vomiting, or diarrhea?

NO → YES → Follow pediatric nausea/vomiting/diarrhea sequence.

2. Is this condition associated with:
   a. abdominal trauma <48 hours?
   b. severe pain?
   c. black or bloody stools?

NO → YES → M.D. STAT

3. Has this condition continued >72 hours?

NO → YES → M.D.

4. Is there:
   a. burning or crying with urination?
   b. frequent urination?

NO → YES → P.A. With urinalysis and culture

P.A.

VS: T, P.

## DYSPHAGIA

Dysphagia means difficulty or pain on swallowing.

1. Dysphagia frequently accompanies a severe sore throat. Make certain that it did not precede or antedate the sore throat. Multiple other causes of dysphagia may require an extensive evaluation by the M.D.

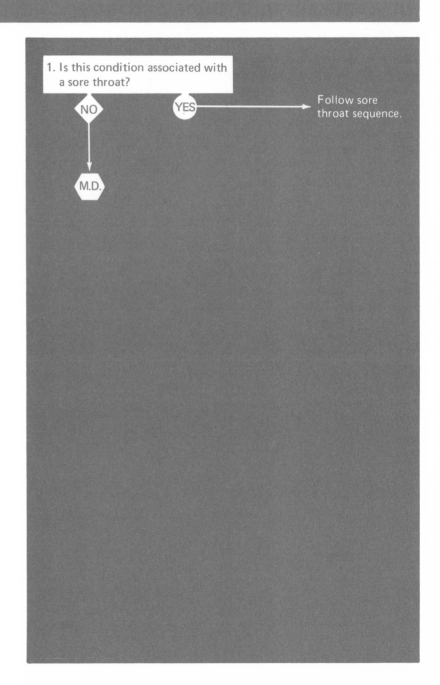

# RECTAL PAIN ● ITCHING

Rectal pain may be interpreted as "fullness," "pressure," or "discomfort." In children, it may be inferred from their actions, e.g., crying with bowel movements or attempted bowel movements.

As always, if the patient is in severe pain, he should be triaged to the M.D. STAT.

Rectal itching is a fairly common complaint with many possible causes. It is triaged in the same manner as rectal pain. It is never so severe as to require triage to the M.D. STAT.

1. Is this associated with rectal bleeding?

NO

YES → Follow rectal bleeding sequence.

M.D.

Associated complaint: Constipation

This flowsheet should be used for all types of rectal bleeding.

1 and 2.  Stools that are black and sticky (like tar) usually represent internal bleeding. "Grossly bloody" stools mean that there is bright red blood in the toilet bowl after each bowel movement. It is often difficult to estimate the amount of blood loss, so bleeding of this type is considered an emergency. In the nonadult, disposition is made to the isolation room because of the possibility of communicable infection.

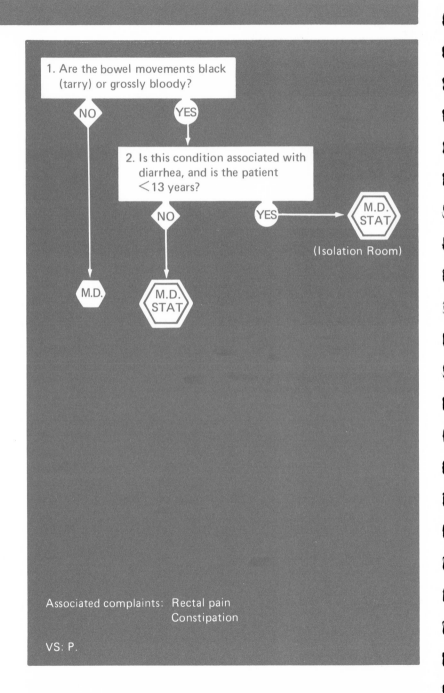

# CONSTIPATION

Constipation is infrequent or difficult bowel movements. However, its meaning to patients may vary widely from painful defecation or narrowing of the caliber of stools, to not having a regular daily bowel movement.

1. Rectal bleeding may occur in several forms: traces of blood on the toilet paper, bright red blood on or mixed with the stool, bright red blood in the toilet, or dark black or tarlike stools. All rectal bleeding should be triaged in the same fashion.

2. In children, pain or difficulty having bowel movements must sometimes be inferred from their behavior, e.g., crying with bowel movements or attempted bowel movements.

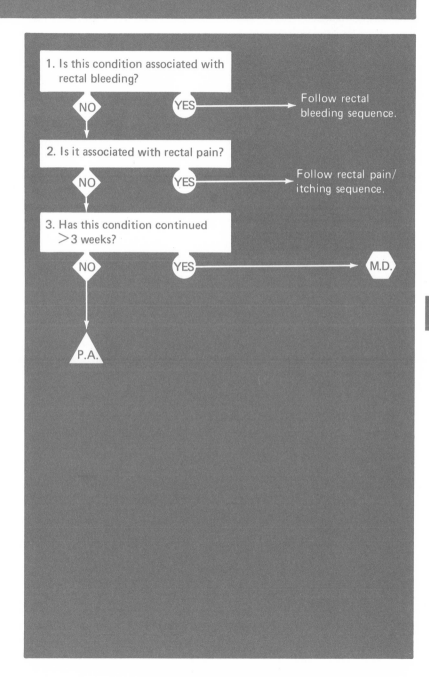

1. Is this condition associated with rectal bleeding?

NO

YES → Follow rectal bleeding sequence.

2. Is it associated with rectal pain?

NO

YES → Follow rectal pain/itching sequence.

3. Has this condition continued >3 weeks?

NO

YES → M.D.

P.A.

## M.D. STAT

1. Nausea, vomiting and/or diarrhea with any of the following:

   a. black and/or bloody vomitus.
   b. severe abdominal pain.
   c. recent (less than forty-eight hours) head trauma.

2. Patients with black and/or bloody stools.

3. Abdominal pain that is severe or associated with black and/or bloody stools or recent (less than forty-eight hours) abdominal trauma.

## M.D.

1. All patients with nausea, vomiting, diarrhea, abdominal pain, or constipation not sent to the M.D. STAT or to the P.A.

2. Rectal pain.

3. Rectal bleeding.

4. Dysphagia not associated with sore throat.

## P.A.

1. Nausea, vomiting and/or diarrhea with *none* of the following:

   a. severe abdominal pain, recent head trauma (less than forty-eight hours), black or bloody stools or vomitus.
   b. duration more than four days (adults); duration more than two days (nonadults).
   c. inability to retain intake more than thirty-six hours (adults); inability to retain intake more than eighteen hours (nonadults).
   d. diabetes.
   e. medications prescribed by the M.D.
   f. temperature more than 101 by history (adults).
   g. more than eight stools a day (adults).
      (VS: T, P, BP.)

2. Abdominal pain (not severe) of less than one-week duration in adults and less than seventy-two hours in nonadults with *no* recent abdominal trauma, black or bloody stools, or possibility of pregnancy.
   (VS: T, P.)

3. Constipation of more than three-weeks duration with *no* rectal pain or rectal bleeding.

54

# GENITOURINARY

## COMPLAINTS

# DYSURIA

Dysuria is pain or burning during urination (voiding, passing water). In the pediatric age group, this problem may be detected if the child cries while urinating (wetting diaper).

1. Shaking chills are defined as episodes of involuntary shaking and teeth chattering associated with cold sensations. This should be distinguished from chilly sensations only. Real shaking chills may indicate septicemia. Vomiting may indicate acute pyelonephritis.

2. If the patient knows he has a kidney disease, an M.D. should handle the problem. Some examples of kidney disease are chronic pyelonephritis (chronic kidney infection), nephrolithiasis (kidney stones) and glomerulonephritis (nephritis). This does *not* include a history of cystitis (bladder infection or urinary tract infection).

3. If there is any question of pregnancy, the triage worker must assume that the answer is "yes." Therefore, the patient should be asked about the *possibility* of pregnancy in a manner that does not convey any moral judgment, regardless of the patient's age or marital status. A matter-of-fact approach is best.

4. Most women have an intermittent discharge consisting of secretions, and it is not a problem to them. This type of discharge is not due to infection. Discharges which *are* due to infection are usually irritating and fairly profuse. Be especially interested in discharges which had their onset in the same general time period as that of the chief complaint.

56

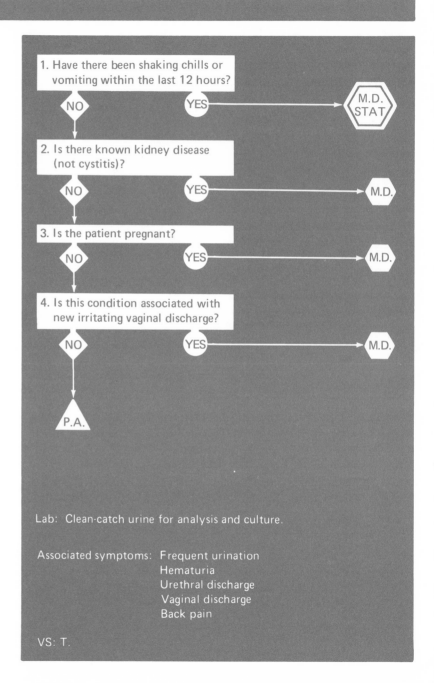

1. Have there been shaking chills or vomiting within the last 12 hours?
NO · YES → M.D. STAT

2. Is there known kidney disease (not cystitis)?
NO · YES → M.D.

3. Is the patient pregnant?
NO · YES → M.D.

4. Is this condition associated with new irritating vaginal discharge?
NO · YES → M.D.

P.A.

Lab: Clean-catch urine for analysis and culture.

Associated symptoms: Frequent urination
Hematuria
Urethral discharge
Vaginal discharge
Back pain

VS: T.

Frequent voiding of small amounts of urine is characteristic of irritation of the bladder by infection. This is usually associated with dysuria. The *total volume* of urine in a given time period will be normal in such a case. In diabetics, however, there is frequent voiding of a normal or even large amount each time. In the case of the diabetic, the problem is not irritation but it is the production of a *total volume* that is larger than normal. This is often associated with thirst as well. To distinguish between urinary tract infection and diabetes, it is important to determine whether the amount voided each time is less than normal, and, thus, indirectly determine whether the total volume of urine is less than normal or more than normal.

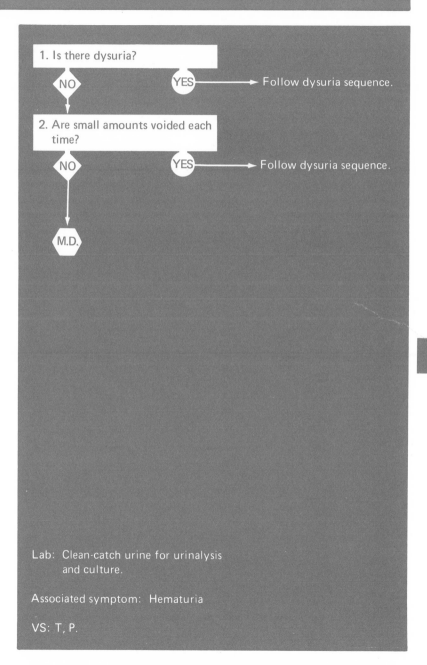

1. Is there dysuria?

NO  YES → Follow dysuria sequence.

2. Are small amounts voided each time?

NO  YES → Follow dysuria sequence.

M.D.

Lab: Clean-catch urine for urinalysis and culture.

Associated symptom: Hematuria

VS: T, P.

57

# HEMATURIA

Hematuria means blood in the urine. Fresh blood will give the urine a pink or red color. Older blood may cause the urine to appear brownish, resembling a cola-type drink. A blood-tinged urethral discharge should be distinguished from hematuria and triaged using the urethral discharge flowsheet.

1. Dysuria is pain or burning on urination (voiding, passing water). In the pediatric age group, it may be detected if the child cries while urinating (wetting diaper).

2. Frequent urination is voiding or passing water more often than normal.

3. A ruptured kidney may not manifest itself until days after it was injured. Any blow or fall that the patient can recall must be considered significant.

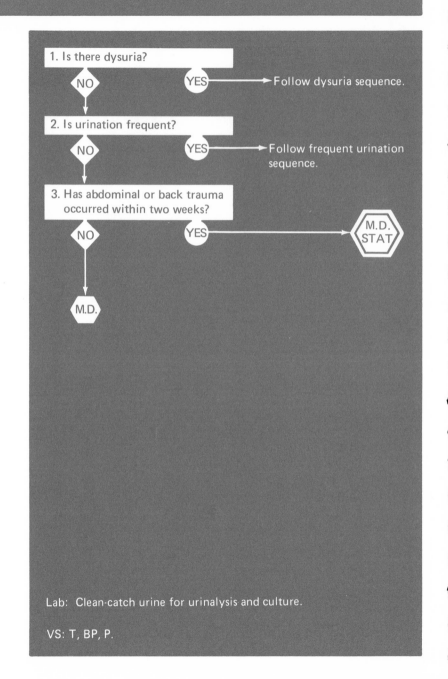

1. Is there dysuria?
NO / YES → Follow dysuria sequence.

2. Is urination frequent?
NO / YES → Follow frequent urination sequence.

3. Has abdominal or back trauma occurred within two weeks?
NO / YES → M.D. STAT

M.D.

Lab: Clean-catch urine for urinalysis and culture.

VS: T, BP, P.

# TESTICULAR PAIN

Testicular pain is pain in the testes, gonads, balls, crotch or however the patient puts it. One cannot be bashful in determining the real site of the pain.

1. Clearly, it is impossible to give a purely quantitative definition of "severe" or "moderate." It is necessary to lean in the direction of overestimation of the severity.

There is usually little difficulty in distinguishing discharge from urine. Discharge is thicker and more opaque than urine. Males may complain of dripping from the penis or say they have the "clap." Females seldom, if ever, identify a urethral discharge as opposed to a vaginal discharge, and it is virtually never identified in children. The discharges may be blood-tinged, and, if so, need to be distinguished from hematuria.

1. Dysuria is pain or burning on urination (voiding, passing water). In the pediatric age group, it may be detected if the child cries while urinating (wetting diaper). Following the dysuria sequence the triage worker will be able to make an appropriate disposition and may avoid problems in the relatively rare cases when urethral discharge is not due to venereal disease.

1. Is there dysuria?

NO

YES → Follow dysuria sequence.

P.A.

Lab: Clean-catch urine for analysis.

VS: T.

## INABILITY TO URINATE

This means the patient is unable to pass any urine or is able to pass only a very small amount of urine occasionally, even with considerable straining. Usually the patient will also complain of discomfort and fullness in the lower abdomen. The disposition is STAT, primarily in the interest of the patient's comfort.

**M.D. STAT**

1. Hematuria without dysuria or frequency and following recent (less than two weeks) back or abdominal trauma.

2. Severe or moderate testicular pain.

3. Patient who is unable to void.

4. Dysuria or frequent small voiding with shaking chills or vomiting within the last twelve hours.

**M.D.**

1. Frequent but not small voiding without dysuria.

2. Mild testicular pain.

3. Dysuria or frequent small voidings with known kidney disease and without vomiting or shaking chills within the last twelve hours.
(VS: T.)

4. Hematuria without dysuria, frequency or recent (within two weeks) abdominal or back trauma.
(VS: T, P, BP.)

5. Dysuria or frequent small voidings with pregnancy.
(VS: T, P, BP.)

6. Dysuria or frequent small voidings with new irritating vaginal discharge.
(VS: T.)

**P.A.**

1. Urethral discharge and dysuria in a male with *no* kidney disease, shaking chills or vomiting within the last twelve hours.
(VS: T.)

2. Urethral discharge in a male without dysuria.
(VS: T.)

3. Dysuria or frequent small voidings with *none* of the following:

   a. shaking chills or vomiting within the last twelve hours.
   b. known kidney disease.
   c. urethral discharge.
   d. new, irritating vaginal discharge.
   e. pregnancy.
   (VS: T.)

## COMPLAINTS

## GYNECOLOGICAL AND BREAST

Unless this is a return visit, *any* problems pertaining to the breast should be triaged using this flowsheet.

2. Severe pain or fever often indicates an infection or abscess which may need to be surgically drained. Such a patient should be evaluated by the M.D.

3. Nursing mothers often have problems with cracked or infected nipples or have difficulty when the child is weaned. The M.D. can advise the patient best, and may possibly prescribe hormone injections.

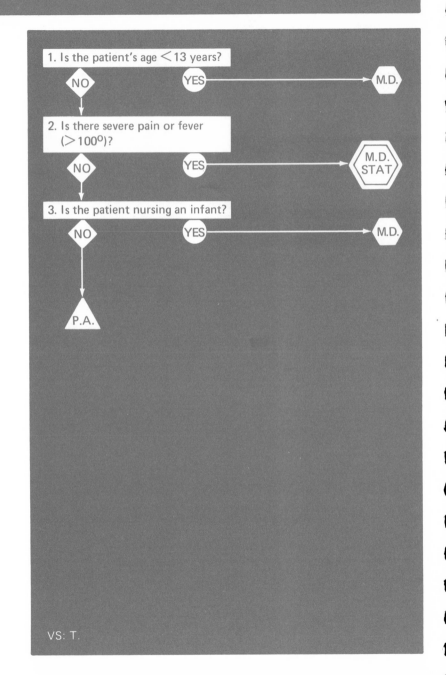

1. Is the patient's age < 13 years?
   - NO
   - YES → M.D.

2. Is there severe pain or fever (> 100°)?
   - NO
   - YES → M.D. STAT

3. Is the patient nursing an infant?
   - NO → P.A.
   - YES → M.D.

VS: T.

## PAP OR ROUTINE PELVIC EXAMINATION

If the patient is requesting this examination because of any symptoms (such as a menstrual problem), then triage should be by the appropriate sequence for that problem.

1. Women who have had abnormal or suspicious Pap tests may be asked to have examinations more frequently; e.g., every three to six months. Otherwise, it is usual to recommend yearly Pap tests on every woman who has not had a complete hysterectomy (uterus and cervix removed) starting in the late teens and continuing for the rest of her life.

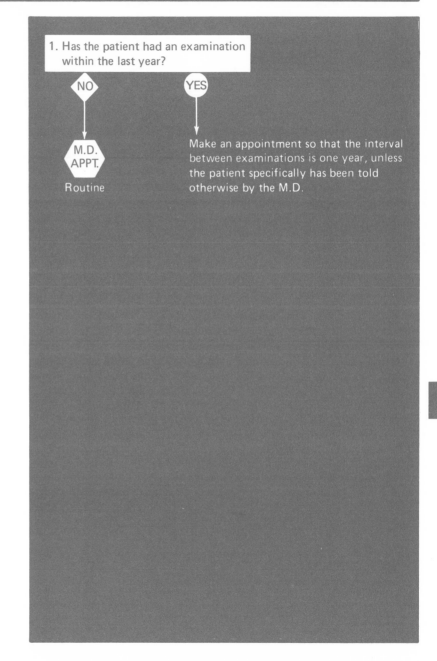

1. Has the patient had an examination within the last year?

NO

YES

M.D. APPT.

Routine

Make an appointment so that the interval between examinations is one year, unless the patient specifically has been told otherwise by the M.D.

## CONTRACEPTIVE OR TUBAL LIGATION REQUEST

Patients desiring birth control or family planning advice or methods will be interviewed concerning the possible use of rhythm, foam, intrauterine device (I.U.D.), birth control pills, or tubal ligation. If the patient is simply requesting a refill of contraceptive prescriptions, then follow medication refill sequence.

M.D. APPT.

Routine

66

1. Present immunologic urine tests for pregnancy are quite accurate, but they still require *at least* forty days since the first day of the last menstrual period before conception occurred. If the patient suspects she is pregnant but had slight bleeding or spotting at the time of her last regular period, she should count the forty days from the time of her last *normal* menstrual period.

   a. If it has not been more than forty days since the patient's last normal menstrual period, she should wait until after forty days and then collect and bring a first voided morning specimen of urine. This is more concentrated and, therefore, more accurate for testing. She can collect an ounce or two in any clean, dry bottle, but it should not sit unrefrigerated for more than three hours.

   b. The patient should be informed when and how she may get results of test.

   c. If two or more periods have been skipped, the patient should be seen by the M.D. regardless of the outcome of the Gravidex. A Gravidex test should be done prior to her appointment.

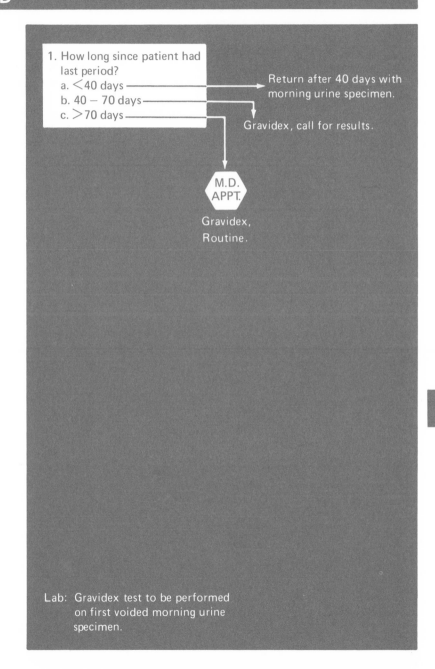

1. How long since patient had last period?
   a. <40 days      Return after 40 days with morning urine specimen.
   b. 40 – 70 days
   c. >70 days      Gravidex, call for results.

M.D. APPT.

Gravidex, Routine.

Lab: Gravidex test to be performed on first voided morning urine specimen.

67

# PREGNANT—APPOINTMENT DESIRED

Unless pregnancy is certain, triage under Missed Period—Pregnancy Suspected.

## PREGNANT—ABORTION DESIRED

Patients desiring therapeutic abortions should be counseled within two or three days. Unless pregnancy is certain, triage under Missed Period—Pregnancy Suspected.

These symptoms are often confused with symptoms of urinary tract infection—frequent, painful or burning urination which should be triaged under frequent urination and dysuria in the genitourinary section. Distinguishing between them can sometimes be a difficult matter, even for the M.D., because of the lack of patient awareness and the personal nature of these complaints.

1 and 2.   If a person has vaginal discomfort, discharge, itching, or irritation, *along with* symptoms suggesting urinary tract infection, she should be triaged according to the dysuria flowsheet. If there is any doubt, use the dysuria flowsheet.

70

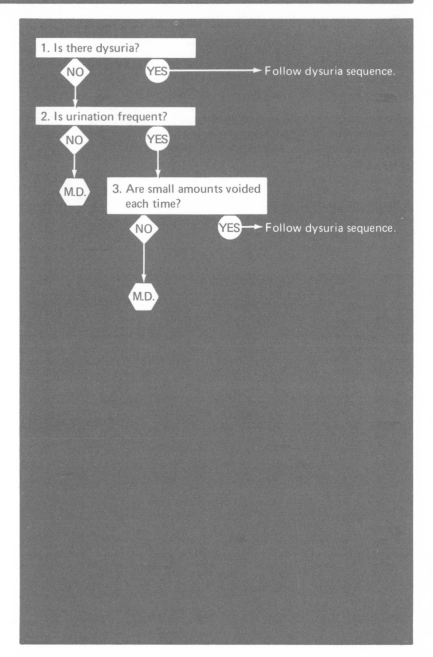

1. Is there dysuria?

NO   YES → Follow dysuria sequence.

2. Is urination frequent?

NO   YES

M.D.   3. Are small amounts voided each time?

NO   YES → Follow dysuria sequence.

M.D.

# VAGINAL BLEEDING

In order to help clarify dispositions for vaginal bleeding, the number of "pads" (sanitary napkins or tampons) used is often obtained. This means the equivalent of fully soaked pads, since many women change pads before they are really saturated with blood.

1. A patient having massive, acute bleeding, or bleeding so brisk that she soaks through more than four pads in an hour should receive prompt attention.

2. Gynecologists feel that a patient using more than ten pads a day, other than on the first day of menses has abnormally heavy bleeding. A fast pulse may also indicate severe bleeding.

3. If this bleeding is during a period that is more than one week late, or if the previous period consisted of only a small amount of spotting, then pregnancy is possible.

4. Any bleeding during the last three months of pregnancy is potentially serious, and the patient should be seen immediately by the M.D. Bleeding in early pregnancy is not uncommon, and if it is a small amount, the patient may be safely seen by the M.D. on a Today basis.

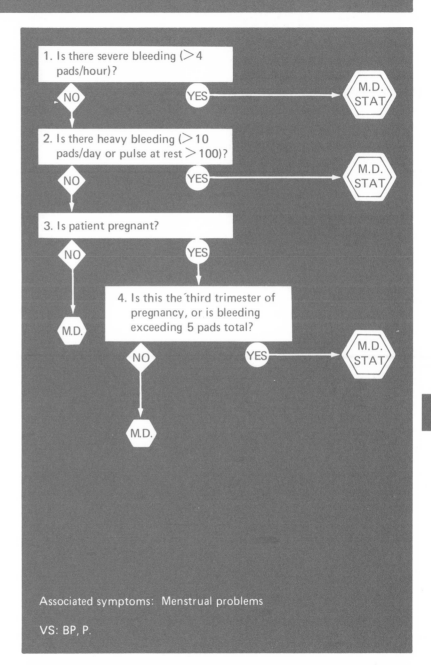

Associated symptoms: Menstrual problems

VS: BP, P.

71

## MENSTRUAL PROBLEMS

This is meant to cover all sorts of menstrual difficulties not covered in other flowsheets. If the problem is a missed period (possible pregnancy), vaginal bleeding, or abdominal pain, it should be triaged according to the appropriate sequence. The most common problems are irregular or painful periods. Any patient who feels she has a problem or difficulties with her periods will be seen by the M.D. This sequence is to help the triage worker decide when a patient should be seen.

1. Discomfort almost always means pain, but also includes moderate or severe anxiety.

2. The problem should not be considered chronic if it has recently become more severe. Most chronic problems are stable or progress very slowly.

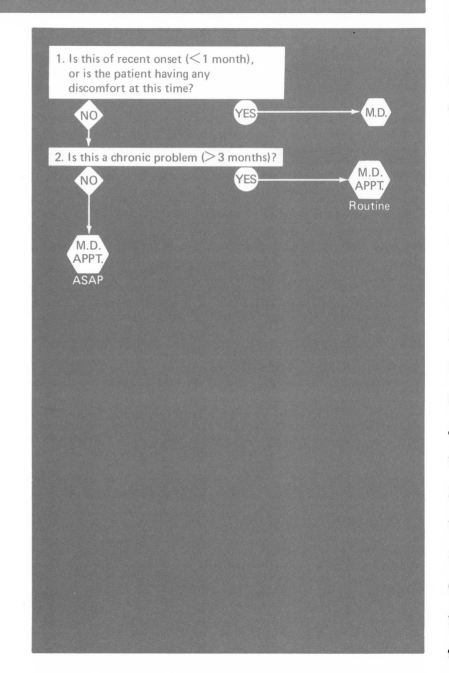

1. Is this of recent onset (< 1 month), or is the patient having any discomfort at this time?

NO → 2. Is this a chronic problem (> 3 months)?

YES → M.D.

NO → M.D. APPT. ASAP

YES → M.D. APPT. Routine

72

## M.D. STAT

1. Heavy vaginal bleeding (more than four pads an hour).

2. Vaginal bleeding of more than five pads total in pregnant patient.

3. Any amount of vaginal bleeding in the third trimester of pregnancy.

4. Breast problems with severe pain or fever (over 100° F).

## M.D.

1. Breast problems in a nursing patient.
(VS: T.)

2. Vaginal discharge, itching, and/or irritation without dysuria or frequent urination.

3. Menstrual problems of recent onset (less than one month) or producing any discomfort, but without *any* of the following:

   a. heavy bleeding (more than ten pads a day).
   b. prolonged bleeding (more than ten days).
   c. patient uncomfortable or pulse at rest of more than 100.
   d. possibility of pregnancy.
   e. pregnancy in first or second trimester or with more than five pads total bleeding.
   (VS: P, BP.)

4. Vaginal bleeding that is not severe (less than four pads an hour) and with *none* of the following:

   a. heavy bleeding (more than ten pads a day).
   b. pregnancy or possible pregnancy.
   c. pulse more than 100 at rest.
   (VS: P, BP.)

## M.D. APPOINTMENT, ASAP

1. Pregnant, abortion desired.

2. Menstrual problems with onset one to three months prior to visit (or getting worse in last three months) and not producing discomfort at this time.

## M.D. APPOINTMENT, ROUTINE

1. Pap or routine pelvic examination request, asymptomatic.

2. Request for contraception.

3. Menstrual problems which are chronic (more than three months) and not getting worse, and patient not having discomfort at this time.

4. Pregnant, appointment desired.

## P.A.

Nonnursing patient with breast problem and *no* severe pain or fever more than 100° F.
(VS: T.)

## COMPLAINTS

# MUSCULO-SKELETAL

This refers to pain along or beside the vertebral column. The pain is confined to the back. If there is soreness at multiple sites, then the patient is probably complaining of diffuse muscle aches, and the muscle aches sequence should be used.

1 and 2. The patient may state that he thinks he injured his back from twisting or straining without direct trauma. If such an injury occurred within the last forty-eight hours, he will be seen in the treatment room by the M.D.

3. (A, B, and C.) In many cases back pain may be associated with urinary tract infections. If there are urinary tract infection symptoms (frequent urination, dysuria, hematuria), the patient's positive answers will lead to the appropriate sequences to be followed.

(D.) If there are abdominal complaints associated with back pain, questions concerning the abdominal pain need to be asked.

4. If this type of back pain has been caused previously by a gynecologic problem, or if the patient thinks a gynecologic problem may be causing this pain, the M.D. should see the patient. Examples of gynecologic problems would be pain with menstrual periods from an ovarian cyst or endometriosis.

5. Many patients will be returning for care of chronic conditions, and they are to be triaged by the appropriate flowsheet. The Medication Refill Request flowsheet will often be required.

76

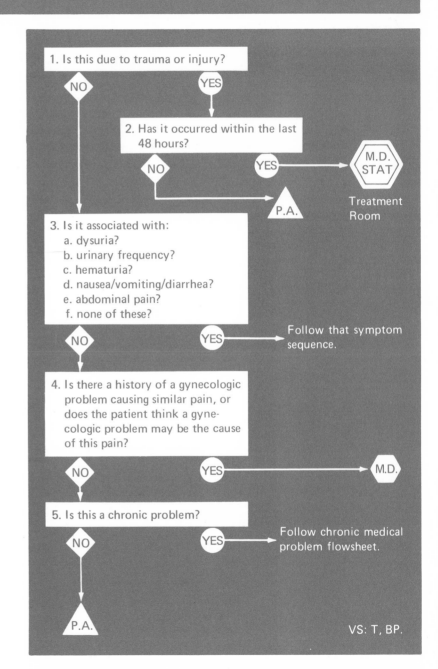

# NECK PAIN

This refers to pain in the back or sides of the neck. Again, if the patient has soreness in other muscles as well, the flowsheet for muscle aches should be followed.

1 and 2.   Neck pain with headache *and* meningismus (stiff neck) warrants emergency evaluation because of the possibility of meningitis.

3. If there is a history of trauma (blow or injury) to the painful area in the past forty-eight hours, the patient should be sent to the treatment room for rapid evaluation by the M.D. Such injury includes twisting or straining of the neck.

4. Many patients will be returning for the care of chronic conditions, and they are to be triaged by the appropriate flowsheet. The Medication Refill Request flowsheet will often be required.

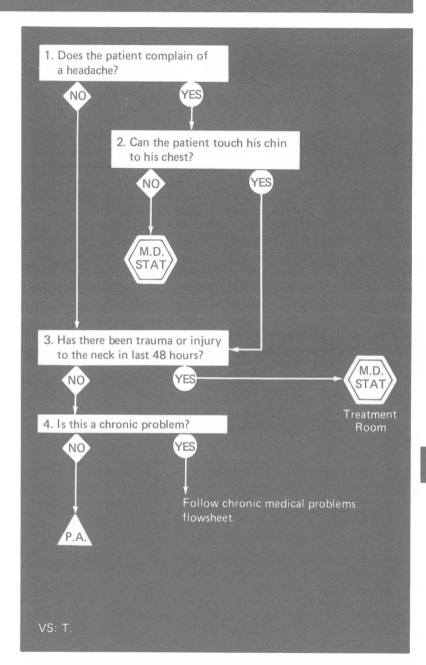

## EXTREMITY PAIN

This flowsheet should be used for any pain in the arm or leg, including pain in the joints of those extremities (shoulder, elbow, hand, finger, hip, knee, ankle, foot, and toe joints). It is difficult to evaluate this complaint without an examination. The P.A. should be able to evaluate adequately most of these problems.

1. If the pain is due to recent trauma, it should be evaluated in the treatment room by the M.D. for possible fracture or joint injury.

2. Many patients will be returning for care of chronic conditions, and they should be triaged by the appropriate flowsheet. The Medication Refill Request flowsheet will often be required.

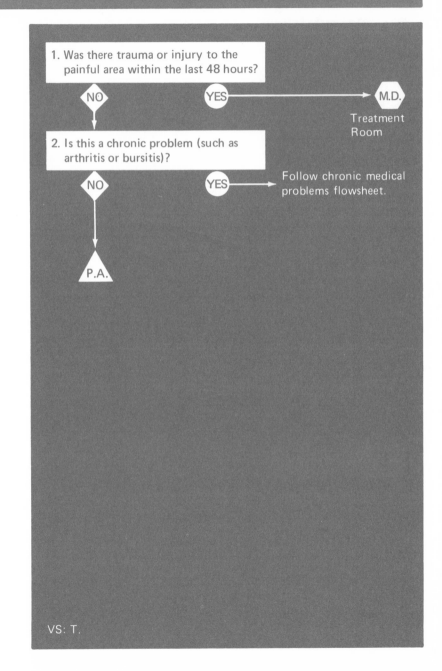

1. Was there trauma or injury to the painful area within the last 48 hours?

NO

YES → M.D. Treatment Room

2. Is this a chronic problem (such as arthritis or bursitis)?

NO

YES → Follow chronic medical problems flowsheet.

P.A.

VS: T.

78

# MUSCLE ACHES (Myalgias)

This is an aching sensation in muscles of the extremities, trunk and/or neck. The most common cause of myalgias is a viral illness. The back muscles are usually most affected, followed by the thigh, neck, shoulder, chest and fine muscles that control the eyeball. Myalgias of the eye muscles cause pain behind the eye whenever the eyes are moved to the extreme right or left.

1 and 2.   Headache is very common in the viral illnesses which produce myalgias. Meningismus, however, is not expected; and, if it is present, meningitis must be ruled out by the M.D. STAT.

3. Myalgias are frequently associated with upper respiratory infections. If the patient has symptoms such as cough, runny nose, sore throat, etc., then follow the appropriate sequence for the correct disposition.

4. Abdominal complaints are not infrequently associated with myalgias. Triaging the primary symptoms will guide the disposition.

5. Sore muscles after overexertion are common, and the patient does not usually seek medical attention for this. Myalgias without overexertion or associated symptoms of a viral illness require evaluation by the M.D.

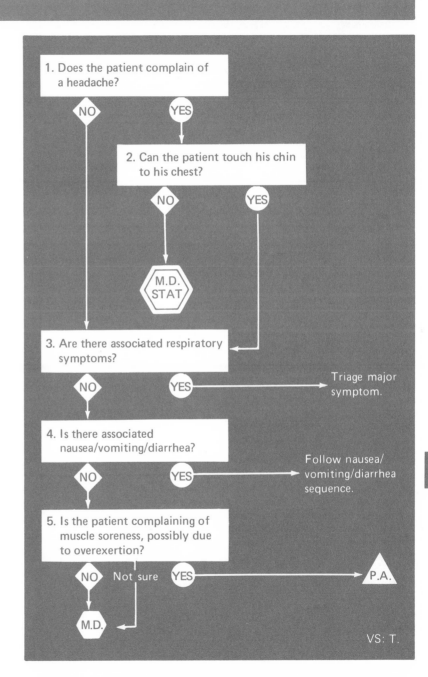

**M.D. STAT**

1. Back or neck pain due to trauma or injury within the last forty-eight hours.

2. Neck pain or myalgias with headache and meningismus (patient unable to touch chin to chest).

**M.D.**

1. Back pain possibly due to a gynecologic problem and with *no* dysuria, frequency, hematuria, nausea, vomiting, diarrhea, or abdominal pain.

2. Muscle aches not due to overexertion and with *no* meningismus, respiratory symptoms, nausea, vomiting, and/or diarrhea.
(VS: T.)

3. Extremity pain (mild or moderate) due to injury within the last forty-eight hours.

**P.A.**

1. Back pain due to trauma or injury that occurred less than forty-eight hours ago.

2. Back pain not due to trauma or a possible gynecologic problem, and with *no* dysuria, frequent urination, hematuria, nausea, vomiting, diarrhea, or abdominal pain.

3. Neck pain without meningismus, and not due to recent (less than forty-eight hours) trauma or injury.

4. Extremity pain not due to recent (less than forty-eight hours) trauma or injury.

5. Muscle aches possibly due to overexertion with *no* meningismus, respiratory symptoms, nausea, vomiting, or diarrhea.

COMPLAINTS

## PODIATRY

A corn is a thickening of the cornified layer which protects the foot. A plantar wart is a wart on the sole of the foot, growing primarily inside the foot with only a small area on the surface. An ingrown toenail extends into the flesh of the toe along its lateral margins. All three may be very painful and may become infected. If the patient is complaining only of foot pain and does not know the cause, the triage worker should triage by following the extremity pain sequence.

1. Patients who are limping from pain or having drainage indicative of infection should be seen by the P.A. on the same day.

2. If the patient is in discomfort with his podiatric problem, he should be seen by the P.A. more quickly than he would be on a routine appointment.

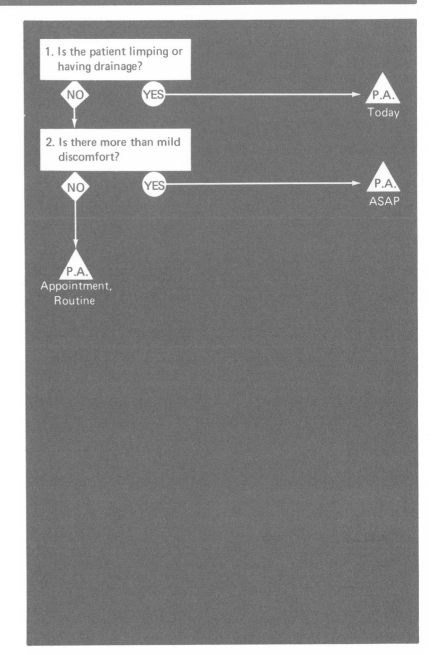

1. Is the patient limping or having drainage?

NO    YES → P.A. Today

2. Is there more than mild discomfort?

NO    YES → P.A. ASAP

P.A. Appointment, Routine

82

**P.A.**

Corns, plantar warts or ingrown toenails with drainage or causing the patient to limp.

**P.A. ASAP**

Corns, plantar warts or ingrown toenails with more than mild discomfort but not causing the patient to limp, and without drainage.

**P.A. APPOINTMENT, ROUTINE**

Corns, plantar warts or ingrown toenails with only mild discomfort and not causing the patient to limp, and without drainage.

83

COMPLAINTS

# DERMATOLOGY

This flowsheet should be used for all skin complaints. Common complaints are acne, alopecia, athlete's foot, boils, burns, dandruff, poison ivy, rash, skin infections, skin lump or growth, skin sore, warts, or any other problem associated with the skin. The ability to make a triage decision by history alone is limited, so the vast majority of these patients are seen by the P.A.

1, 2, 3, and 4.   These are the only dispositions that reliably can be made on history alone.

5. A skin problem with fever may be an urgent situation and should be seen by the M.D.

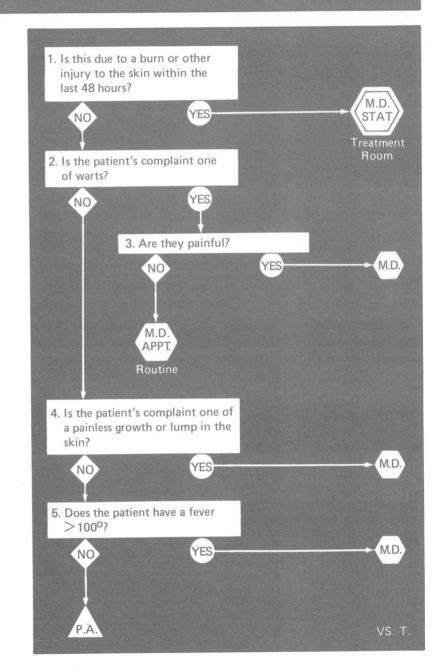

86

VS: T.

**M.D. STAT**

Burn or injury to skin in the last forty-eight hours.

**M.D.**

1. Painful warts.

2. Painless growth or lump in skin.

3. Any skin problem with a fever (over 100).

**M.D. APPOINTMENT, ROUTINE**

Painless warts.

**P.A.**

All skin problems not covered by the above criteria.
(VS: T.)

## COMPLAINTS

## MISCELLANEOUS

## MEDICATION REFILL REQUEST

1. If there are any questions about clinical problems, the physician should evaluate them.

2. The P.A. should expedite refill requests by identifying those which can be documented in the patient's record.

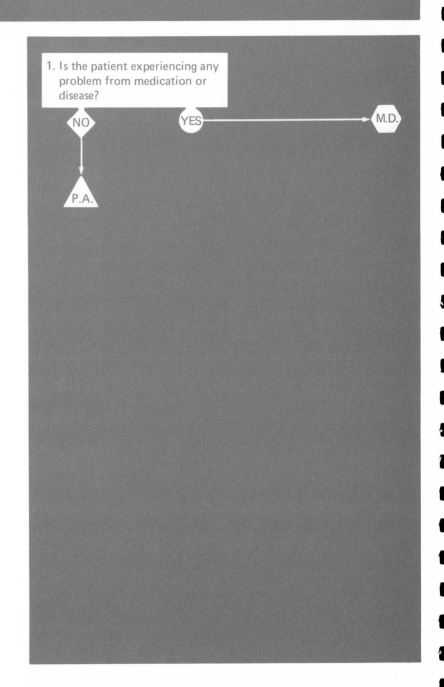

## VASECTOMY REQUEST

Men desiring sterilization by vasectomy (cutting of the tubes leading from the testicles to the penis) may make a routine appointment for discussion of the procedure.

## BEE STING OR INSECT BITE

Patients with acute stings or bites are sent to the treatment room because of the possibility of severe allergic manifestations requiring potent drugs and/or injections.

1. Severe and potentially lethal allergic reactions may occur and are characterized by choices *a* through *c*. (See cardiorespiratory and dermatology sections for descriptions of those problems.) Severe local reactions may also occur, especially following a spider or poisonous insect bite.

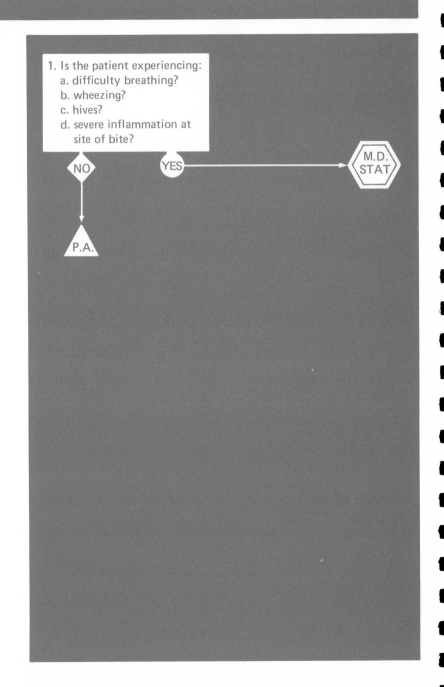

1. Is the patient experiencing:
   a. difficulty breathing?
   b. wheezing?
   c. hives?
   d. severe inflammation at site of bite?

NO — P.A.

YES — M.D. STAT

## SPONTANEOUS RETURN FOR CURRENT EPISODE OF ILLNESS

A spontaneous return is a visit by a patient who was seen recently for a problem but not told to return for further followup at this time. The patient may be returning because the problem is not improving or because of anxiety or misunderstanding.

It is always advisable for a patient to return to the same care provider who had seen him the first time. Every patient returning to see the P.A. should be checked by the M.D. to be sure that no medical error is made.

Return patient to the medical provider who last saw him.

## CARE PROVIDER REQUEST FOR PATIENT'S RETURN

Make a routine appointment with the provider requesting patient's return, unless a different provider was specified.

To appropriate care provider.

94

## SUTURE REMOVAL

All patients returning for routine suture removal should be triaged directly to the P.A.

1. It is important to identify the patient who desires a physical examination as a way of dealing with symptoms as opposed to the patient who wants a screening examination for employment, etc.

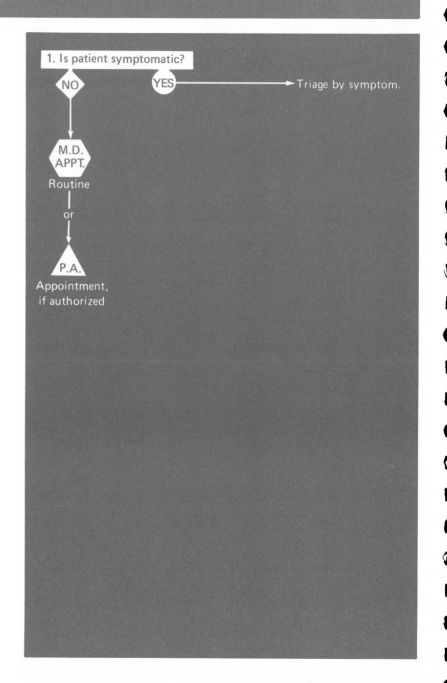

1. Is patient symptomatic?

NO

YES → Triage by symptom.

M.D. APPT.
Routine

or

P.A.
Appointment,
if authorized

# CHRONIC MEDICAL PROBLEM

This flowsheet is designed to effect appropriate disposition for patients with established medical problems that require chronic follow-up care. Such problems include hypertension, heart disease, diabetes, arthritis, gout, seizure disorders, asthma or other chronic lung disease, cirrhosis or other chronic liver disease, and chronic kidney disease. Many of these patients have not been followed regularly and are in need of establishing contact with a physician who will emphasize the need for regular monitoring as well as self-care. These diseases cannot be adequately followed on an episodic basis.

1. If the patient's major problem is with his medications, he should be seen by the M.D. so that his treatment will not be interrupted while awaiting an appointment.

2. There is a real advantage to the clinic and to the patient to be seen by appointment rather than as a walk-in. If, however, the patient reports that his condition has been worsening recently, he will need to be seen more promptly.

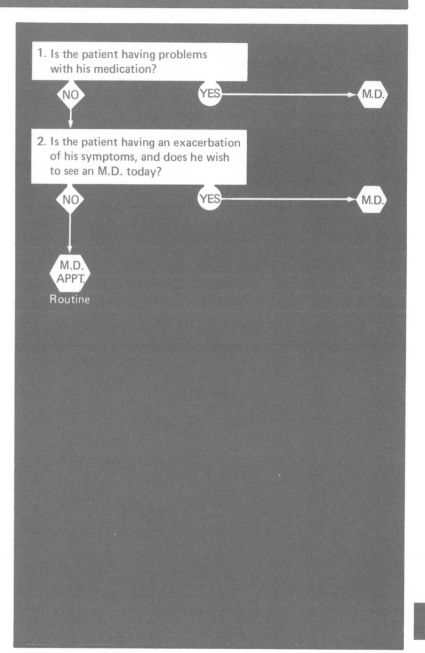

1. Is the patient having problems with his medication?

NO   YES → M.D.

2. Is the patient having an exacerbation of his symptoms, and does he wish to see an M.D. today?

NO   YES → M.D.

M.D. APPT.
Routine

# BLOOD PRESSURE CHECK

This flowsheet should be used only for those people whose blood pressure is being recorded for diagnostic purposes. Patients who have hypertension and want their blood pressure checked and medicines refilled should be triaged under Chronic Medical Problems and Medication Refill Request.

## LABORATORY WORK REQUEST

The P.A. may perform or order lab work required for employment or a marriage license or previously authorized by an M.D. Requests for other reasons will need the approval of the M.D.

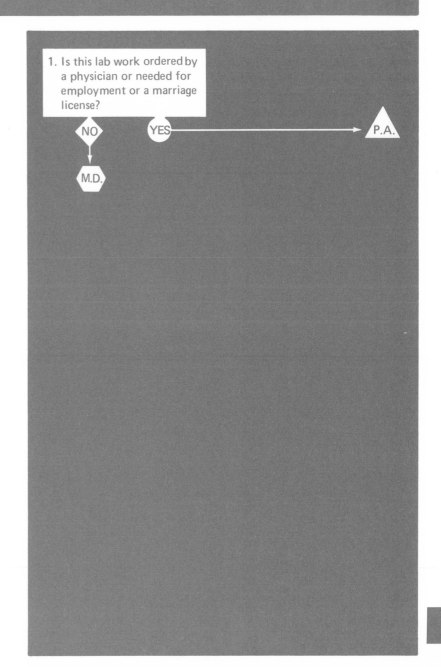

## COMPLAINT NOT ON LIST

The M.D. will speak with the triage worker and/or the patient to decide the most appropriate disposition.

### M.D. STAT

1. Bee sting or insect bite with difficulty breathing, wheezing, hives or a severe local reaction.

### M.D.

1. Medication refill request and problems with medication or disease.

2. Any complaint not listed in this manual.

3. Return requested by the physician.

4. Spontaneous return, last seen by the physician.

5. Chronic disease, problems with disease or medications.

6. Lab work, not for employment or marriage license.

### M.D. APPOINTMENT, ROUTINE

1. Vasectomy request.

2. Routine examination or checkup.

3. Chronic disease, no problems with disease or medications.

### P.A.

1. Nonacute bee sting or insect bite occurring more than twenty-four hours ago.

2. Medication refill request, no unexpected problems with medication or disease.

3. Return requested by P.A.

4. Spontaneous return, last seen by P.A.

5. Suture removal.

6. Blood pressure check.

7. Lab work for employment or marriage license.

# INDEX OF COMPLAINTS